# Ethical Issues in Palliative Care

## Second Edition

**Edited by**

## Patricia Webb

*Principal Lecturer in Cancer and Palliative Care*
*St George's Hospital Medical School*
*Editor, European Journal of Cancer Care*

**Foreword by**

## Ian Ainsworth-Smith

Radcliffe Publishing
Oxford ● Seattle

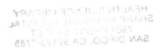

**Radcliffe Publishing Ltd**
18 Marcham Road
Abingdon
Oxon OX14 1AA
United Kingdom

www.radcliffe-oxford.com
Electronic catalogue and worldwide online ordering facility.

First edition 2000 (published by Hochland & Hochland Ltd)

British Library Cataloguing in Publication Data

A catalogue record for this book is available from the British Library.

ISBN 1 85775 825 0

Typeset by Acorn Bookwork Ltd, Salisbury, Wiltshire
Printed and bound by TJ International Ltd, Padstow, Cornwall

# Contents

# Foreword

I am delighted to offer the Foreword for this new edition. It is at first sight surprising that a new edition of this book should be needed within five years of its original publication and successful reception. This revised edition, however, reflects fully the changes that have taken place in palliative care practice and in ethical thinking over a relatively short period. It should serve as a reminder that ethics always takes place in context. The context has been formed in part by changing and developing expectations on the part of patients, those close to them who may also seek to act as their advocates, the general public and health-care professionals. It would have been remarkable if palliative care textbooks written a decade ago had contained a developed discussion of the need for resuscitation policies and protocols in palliative care! The boundary between 'palliative' and 'curative' care will continuously rearrange itself in line with increasing possibilities in clinical care. Research is now undertaken regularly with the aim of developing improved palliative care. It is of great importance but self-evidently requires thoughtful and ethically rigorous critique.

This book reminds us that 'ethical' and 'legal' issues are related but do not, and should not, always converge. In the United Kingdom and elsewhere the courts have been increasingly called upon to give an opinion on 'end of life' cases where there is genuine and apparently irreconcilable divergence of opinion between the patient, those who seek to offer advocacy and those responsible for the patient's care. In these circumstances staying inside the requirements of the law may become confused with optimal ethical practice. The 'best interests' of the patient may not be the immediate medical need.

Some texts on medical ethics which deal with palliative care may be quite 'unrooted' in practice or be so concerned with the individual case that they may run the risk of 'special pleading'. The overriding principle of good ethical practice must be to help pose the right questions, open the 'what if' scenario and not to seek 'correct' answers precipitately. This book's strength is that it encourages the reader to consider a particular situation and to identify the process by which a course of action is reached.

The authors' diverse professional backgrounds lead them to develop their case but also to acknowledge that theirs may not be the only contribution to the debate. In the original Foreword it was hoped that the reader would be challenged, helped or even outraged. In this book's updated form, that task continues to be developed. Familiar territory is re-covered, new questions are asked and the outline of debates which may follow in the future is left for the reader to take forward. If that takes place, this book will fully have served its purpose.

Ian Ainsworth-Smith
Chaplain, St George's Healthcare NHS Trust
Chairman, St George's Hospital Clinical Ethics Committee
Vice-Chairman, South-East Multicentre Research Ethics Committee
Honorary Canon, Southwark Cathedral
*April 2005*

# Preface

Like the first edition of this book, the following is not meant to be a definitive text about palliative care ethics. It is intentionally a collection of reflections and ideas from a variety of professionals with a vested interest in the subject as well as a personal one. They have either worked in palliative care in the past or are doing so now. They are teaching or researching aspects of palliative care, or come into regular contact with patients and families who have life-limiting, progressive illness – or all of the above.

All of us who have contributed to this book acknowledge the difficulties in making ethical decisions in the everyday practice of palliative care. All of us acknowledge that in theory a multi-professional approach to such decision making is helpful. This second edition includes more ideas about decision making and models for the latter. Over the years we have tried to help each other in a variety of ways, not least by discussing some of the thorny issues for all clinicians and the patients with whom they work. Since the publication of the first edition there have been some real and controversial issues discussed in palliative care, and some national debates on aspects of it. Certain of these are helpfully included in this book.

As the specialty of palliative care becomes more sophisticated and the illness trajectories of patients become longer, the ethical issues are changing. They also change because societies change – in their values, views, beliefs and the degree of involvement in decisions related to health and illness. Palliative care is now not just about the end stage of diseases like cancer and motor-neuron disease, but includes *all* illnesses that are currently non-curable and life-limiting. Palliative care is also about long and short patient trajectories. The pattern for some multiple sclerosis sufferers is very different from that for patients with far-advanced chronic obstructive pulmonary disease. A palliative care patient may be looking at 20 years of life with infrequent exacerbations of their illness, or they may be looking at a rapid decline to death. Because of these changes in the specialty, a whole range of new ethical issues have arisen and will continue to do so. For those working in generalist settings, the implementation of palliative care standards and ideals may be more difficult to achieve, and having like minds to consider an ethical issue more demanding. It is hoped that this book will aid health professionals in consultation with others whether within or outside their own units or care settings.

It is frequently claimed that there are no finite or absolute answers to ethical dilemmas. The contributors to this book have therefore raised questions, debated them, and on some occasions given their own opinion but, more helpfully, they have also left the reader with some tools to enable him or her to think in a more structured and rational way about dilemmas.

Many of the issues covered in this book are raised regularly by the health professionals of tomorrow – including undergraduate and postgraduate students from a variety of programmes as well as those who are taking time out to professionally update. Others have been hotly debated by current practitioners who work on a daily basis in a specialist palliative care setting or in a more general one, whether in institutions or in patients' own homes.

All of the contributors to this book are well used to teaching health professionals (or aspiring students of different professional disciplines) in mixed groups. In our collective experience this is by far the most useful way of teasing out real dilemmas and rehearsing as yet unexplored ones. Group members do of course approach dilemmas from their own professional stance, but with the recognition that theirs is not the sole contribution to be made.

To say that we all need all of the help that we can muster would not be exaggerating the point. If patients and families are to be helped to understand what is happening to them and to be given a balanced view of some of the difficult ethical decisions they will have to make in their alliance or contract with those who are caring for them, they need to have confidence that expertise is available. They need to know that ethics is a taught subject which is deliberated by a range of professionals. These may be moral philosophers, clergy, doctors, nurses, physiotherapists, radiographers – or whoever. Combining the expertise has in our view been helpful.

We all very much hope that you will be challenged, helped or even outraged if it enables us all to present a more rational and balanced view of ethics in everyday palliative care.

Patricia Webb
*April 2005*

# List of contributors

**Rachel Burman**
Palliative Medicine Consultant
Department of Palliative Care and Policy
Guy's, King's and St Thomas' School of Medicine
King's College London

**Heather Draper** PhD
Senior Lecturer in Biomedical Ethics
Centre for Biomedical Ethics
University of Birmingham

**Calliope Farsides**
Senior Lecturer in Medical Ethics
Centre of Law and Medical Ethics
King's College London

**David Jeffrey**
Retired Palliative Medicine Consultant
Chair of Ethics Committee
Association for Palliative Medicine
Great Britain and Ireland

**Marney Prouse** LLM, RN
Consultant in Risk and Quality
Formerly, Quality Assurance Advisor
Trinity Hospice and Palliative Care
Evaluation Lead
King's Fund/Macmillan Cancer Relief

**Robert Stanley**
Senior Lecturer in Ethics
Faculty of Health and Social Care Sciences
Kingston University

**Patricia Webb**
Principal Lecturer in Cancer and Palliative Care
St George's Hospital Medical School
Editor, *European Journal of Cancer Care*

**Roger Worthington** PhD
Standards and Ethics Advisor
General Medical Council

# 1 Why is the study of ethics important?

## Patricia Webb

## Introduction

The study of ethics and the study and practice of healthcare have not merged much in the past, but nevertheless ethical standards are essential to the practice of the health professions. Each professional discipline has its own code of conduct, guidelines for practice and philosophy of care to direct practice within its professional remit. There have been several international declarations of human rights within healthcare to protect patients from unethical practices that might nevertheless be portrayed to them as necessary evils in the course of scientific research and utilitarian principles – that is, the greater good.

Despite the relative lack of moral philosophy and healthcare ethics in the curricula of healthcare professionals, it does not take long for anyone in clinical practice to face their first ethical dilemma about which they are called upon to make a judgement or have a view.

In any healthcare system, whether organised and managed by the state or government or by the independent sector (private or non-governmental/voluntary) – or any mixture of these – moral issues will frequently be raised and should challenge the practitioner, teacher, manager or researcher. Establishing moral codes of practice between the various organisations mentioned above is important at the outset of any professional relationship or client encounter.

For the practitioner the appropriate use of professional power, compared with the relative vulnerability of the lay client/patient during the first meeting, establishes the relationship for all future transactions between the two parties. In the context of progressive illness there are many occasions that will challenge this relationship as the illness trajectory takes its course. There are increasing numbers of situations which pose ethical dilemmas, whether it be in the equal allocation of resources, equal accessibility to healthcare services, decisions about the right treatments or best care, or the right to life or to end life. All of these examples raise the so-called 'classic' ethical principles of justice or fairness, autonomy, beneficence and non-maleficence[1,2] (*see* Chapter 2 for an alternative way of looking at issues).

Some health carers may have studied moral philosophy as part of their general education or pursued it as a personal interest, while others may have no grounding at all in this subject. In either case, applying moral philosophy to the real world of work with patients in health services, driven by political and/or financial agendas, is difficult. It is equally difficult in those health services which are managed partly by the state and partly by private insurers, or indeed those which are managed by the independent sector, whether non-governmental organisations or private companies. All have vested interests, and all have their own agendas.

'Justice for all' is an easy phrase to use, but how does one decide whether, for example, a young woman with breast cancer, whose only apparent chance of survival (and possibly cure) is an expensive course of drugs, or a young child with cystic fibrosis, whose only chance of survival is a heart–lung transplant, should be allocated the resources from a finite pot when there is money for only one of these two? How can provision be made to satisfy a palliative care patient's autonomy to remain in their own home, when the only way to achieve this is to enlist the support of a reluctant and unco-operative relative to act as the main carer, and again to find the financial resources for professional backup and support?

# Professional education and training

Apart from the knowledge base of moral philosophy, the most important function of studying ethics is to encourage logical, reasoned thinking rather than an unreasoned 'knee-jerk' reaction to a given situation in everyday work.

In medical practice the code of medical conduct – the Hippocratic oath – which used to be sworn by newly qualified doctors was reinforced by the more recent international codes and declarations formulated as a result of disregard for human rights through human experimentation and sometimes violation.

These codes include the Nuremberg Code and the Geneva Convention in the 1940s, and the Declaration of Helsinki in the 1960s, amended in the 1970s, which was followed by discussion on national codes of ethical medical practice in the USA and Europe, and the development of the Institute of Human Values in Medicine in the USA. Details of all of these can be found in the text and appendices of several publications, one of which is by Campbell *et al.*[3] The deficit in the teaching of ethics to doctors resulted in the British Medical Association in 1986 calling for all UK medical schools to provide substantial medical ethics and human values teaching, and in the recommendations of the General Medical Council (GMC) that the doctors of tomorrow need to receive such education.[4] Medical ethics is now part of the regular medical curriculum in several countries, including the USA and the UK.

Apart from doctors, other healthcare professionals also have their own codes of conduct or guidelines for practice, which include acknowledging the human rights of relatively vulnerable patients and being aware of their own professional responsibilities and duty to care. They, too, now have some regular input on ethics as it applies to healthcare in their first-level training and in continuous professional development at all academic levels.

However, codes of conduct and guidelines for practice are only part of the story. They provide some parameters within which to work, but they do not necessarily guide one's thinking through an ethical dilemma (such as those already quoted above) to encourage formulation of a viewpoint or judgement.

# Clinical trials

Much of the debate on ethical issues in healthcare has been related to the inclusion of human subjects in clinical trials, primarily for cancer and aspects of psychiatry research. The majority of ethics committees were originally established to scrutinise research protocols for these trials. International protocols have to be seen and agreed by the national and local ethics committees before each of the countries involved can sign up to the trial, and before the final scan for ethical practice by the relevant pharmaceutical company. In the UK, some of the regional and, to an even greater extent, local ethics committees have extended their roles to consider other kinds of research proposals to ensure appropriate ethical practice, but these are currently still in the minority, and are by no means available in all regions.

# Research ethics

Consideration needs to be given to the ethical issues involved in all of the elements of research, not just those for human experimentation. These include choosing the appropriate methods for conducting the research, the choice of an appropriate sample, the issue of inclusion of patients and/or their relatives, confidentiality for the research subjects, adequate funding and resourcing to complete the work, and so on. All of these are important considerations for the researcher.

# Palliative care

What does all of this have to do with the practice of palliative care? Clinical trials have only just begun in this specialty, and other research has been slow to develop. Palliative care is still an emerging specialty, and is only now adding to the earlier successes of systematic investigation into pain management and the early studies on bereavement. Now a wide range of issues are the subjects of research through the use of either quantitative or qualitative methods, or a combination of these.

The reasons given for not establishing an evidence base for palliative care earlier were sometimes muddled and sometimes realistic. It was considered that any research involving the seriously ill or dying was intensely intrusive. There was some justification for this view, but some people who were facing imminent death would have been pleased to share even that intensely private and lonely experience with those who were keen to learn from it. Systematic investigation of people's feelings, symptoms, anxiety levels and life quality are all now included in research topics. Intrusion into a patient's life is still recognised as a potential problem, but great care can be taken in the design of research to counter or minimise this and to gain appropriate compliance from some patients.

Attrition rates can pose a greater problem in palliative care compared with other specialties and have to be considered carefully as part of the research design. One way of minimising the effects of this is to extend the sample size by collaboration between several centres rather than undertaking more parochial and local research projects. Other standard statistical considerations also need to be taken into account – for example, appropriate sample sizes for the number of variables. With palliative care services being offered much earlier in the illness trajectory, some of these issues are less problematic than they once were. Patients may live longer than the terminal care patient of just a few decades ago, and their illness may be less traumatic because of improvements in symptom management and control.

Patients have not been the only subjects of research. Carers have also played a very significant part in adding to the palliative care knowledge base, particularly in the areas of loss and bereavement and of caring.[5]

# Ethics in practice

There are many instances in the everyday practice of palliative care, rather than the research into it, when decisions have to be made that include ethical, clinical and practical issues. Any or all of four ethical principles considered appropriate to healthcare may need to be considered and debated. These four principles are beneficence, non-maleficence, autonomy and justice. An ethical viewpoint is not just a matter of opinion, but requires reasoned and rational thinking in order to propose several possible solutions to a dilemma, and then to find the most appropriate one in the circumstances, using these four principles as a basis for the reasoning. However, it must be acknowledged that opinions differ on the use of the four principles (*see* Chapters 2 and 3).

# Justice

For example, in the case of justice, is it just to respect and provide what are seen as a person's rights – in this context, good palliative care services – in the knowledge that, at least in a democracy, a person has the right to medical treatment and healthcare? If so, what if there are only sufficient resources for one person when two individuals require them simultaneously?

Should justice be interpreted as what someone feels that they deserve or need – rather than necessarily their right? In the former case one could easily be trapped into the meritocracy argument. For example, consider a person who has never smoked a cigarette and yet has developed lung cancer. Should he have the best treatment for his cancer, rather than the person who has smoked cigarettes all his life? Another example may be the question of whether to give treatment or allocate resources to someone who is still able to contribute economically to society, compared with a physically or mentally disabled person or someone of older age who has less chance of demonstrating such a contribution.

In considering needs, should those who have the most perceived needs – the poor, the sick and the socially disadvantaged – receive first, before those who are privileged, despite having similar medical requirements?

# Justice and autonomy

There is much rhetoric given to the notion of autonomy in today's consumer society. Justice – rights and responsibilities – is often portrayed as 'I' have rights and 'you' have the responsibility to provide for them, rather than the two in balance. Patients' rights have been the subject of much recent discussion, perhaps in an attempt to redress the many years of paternalism which was little short of coercion at times. That said, there are some positive aspects of paternalism which still sometimes have a place in healthcare.

Although in the palliative care setting patients have some moral rights (to fair and equal treatment and care, to privacy and confidentiality, to autonomy and to information and truth), they also have some responsibilities.

If a contractual alliance to plan care together is established between patient and professional, then there are responsibilities to fulfil on both sides of the alliance. One could frequently argue that satisfying one patient's rights may infringe the rights of another patient, relative or health professional. A clear example of this is the current cry of a 'patient's right to die' when they may wish the professional to help them to end their life, and they therefore run the risk of implicating them in their death. This can be seen as an infringement of the professional's right to practise his or her profession properly and legally. A whole chapter is devoted to this particular issue later in this book (*see* Chapter 7).

# Doing good (beneficence)

As was mentioned earlier, systematic research on all aspects of palliative care is a relatively recent activity. The evidence for doing good has in the past relied on anecdotes or letters of thanks to those providing palliative care services. Although these are not to be discounted, the introduction of standards against which to measure 'doing good' is to be welcomed. Gratitude for being in a comfortable or comforting environment is one achievement of palliative care provision, but that alone may not provide the best quality of life possible for an individual with palliative care needs.[6] They need to know what may be possible if they are to ask for it.

# Doing harm (maleficence)

What is the definition and meaning of 'harm'? If the whole ethos of palliative care is to make the very best of the life that is left, then the relative risks and benefits of all proposed treatment and care need to be considered by the patient (with or without their relatives, as they wish) and the professional carers. There is frequently considerable disagreement about what constitutes 'harm' for an individual. The disagreement may be between two health professionals. For example, pain may be perceived by doctor or nurse 'A' to be the cause of most harm to patient X. Morphine should be given to relieve it, despite its sometimes unwanted effects on the central nervous system of initial drowsiness and impaired concentration (which could also be caused by the pain itself). A second doctor or nurse, 'B', may consider that although pain is present and in their view is causing harm, there are less effective analgesics than morphine, but ones that would limit the unwanted effects on the central nervous system. Pain would be reduced but not eliminated, and concentration and alertness would be retained. The partially relieved pain may itself arguably impair concentration to some extent, but not so much as the effects of morphine would do. What are the relative benefits and risks with regard to quality of life for such a patient?

Then consider the patient's perspective. He does not perceive his pain as the worst harm. He is a practising academic and wants to continue working despite his serious illness. Work is his main *raison d'être*. He wants to drink alcohol to relieve his pain (which he is well used to doing). For him it partly relieves his pain, it makes him relaxed (which also helps to reduce the pain) and, because of his tolerance to it, he retains a sharp, incisive mind to continue his work.

This example causes a problem for professionals. Although alcohol may be taken in moderation, the amounts that this patient is used to would be considered by them to be harmful. They know what will do good in reducing the patient's pain, but they are torn between their convictions and the need to respect the patient's autonomy.

# Conclusions

So why is it important to study ethics, particularly in relation to palliative care? Clearly there are ethical issues and dilemmas to be considered every day in palliative care, just as there are clinical ones. The two really are inseparable. The decision to rehydrate a patient in the last days of life has both clinical implications and ethical ones. The decision to retain a seriously ill patient in an inpatient unit for care because there are inadequate support services in their own home to deal with the extent of difficult symptoms (despite their own wish to be at home) poses clinical as well as ethical issues. Each individual human story is complex and frequently difficult to resolve at all levels. Each situation needs to be considered in a logical, objective way as well as an emotional, human one. Then a balanced view needs to be taken, preferably jointly with more than one professional who knows the circumstances, and in dialogue with family members if that is desired by the patient.

The study of ethics is important to enable such reasoning to take place in the context of an understanding of the moral issues that are part of all of our practice. Several innovative ways of teaching ethics have been proposed and tried in palliative care. It is well worth looking at these models from the literature. It is also valuable to search for models of teaching ethics in other specialties, with a view to replicating them in the care of the seriously ill. Much has already been successfully achieved.

In addition to the theoretical input of educational programmes on applied moral philosophy, Burman (*see* Chapter 8) has addressed the teaching of ethics in the practice setting for palliative care. There is no doubt that simulating hypothetical examples of frequently occurring ethical dilemmas for use in teaching (particularly multi-professional teaching) is extremely valuable. Extending these ideas into 'rehearsing' real situations that are likely to occur for individual patients is also helpful. Anticipating potential dilemmas and discussing them with other professional colleagues is helpful in planning for the real event, when time may well be against one.

The study of ethics is every bit as important as the study of each individual's main professional discipline – be it medicine, nursing, religion, social work, or whatever. In this crucial time in a patient's life, when life itself is limited and under threat (and you have warning of that, compared with sudden death), every opportunity should be taken to reason with them the best path to tread for all concerned. There will never be one right answer to an ethical dilemma, just a series of possible solutions from which to select the most appropriate for all concerned.

# References

1 Beauchamp T and Childress J (1983) *Biomedical Ethics*. Oxford University Press, Oxford.
2 Doyle D, Cherny NI and Calman KC (2004) *Oxford Textbook of Palliative Medicine*. Section 3. Oxford University Press, Oxford.
3 Campbell A, Charlsworth M, Gillett G and Jones G (1997) *Medical Ethics*. Oxford University Press, Auckland.
4 General Medical Council (1996) *Tomorrow's Doctors*. General Medical Council, London.
5 Seale C and Cartwright A (1994) *The Year Before Death*. Avebury Press, Aldershot.
6 Addington-Hall J and Higginson I (2001) *Palliative Care for Non-Cancer Patients*. Oxford University Press, Oxford.

# 2 Critical decision making: moving from theory to practice

## Roger Worthington

## Introduction

The conceptual basis for the making of difficult decisions is a complex and intriguing topic of philosophical discussion. In the context of applied ethics, careful analysis is needed to identify the basis upon which critical decisions are made. Theories of decision making vary greatly and encompass domains ranging all the way from logic, mathematics and game theory to jurisprudence and democratic justice. However, this chapter aims not so much to be comprehensive in terms of propositional theory as to try to explore the conceptual basis upon which an ethical framework for practical decision making can be built. When the issues concern matters of life and death and questions of fundamental values and choice, as in the case of ethics and palliative care, they demand serious consideration.

It is a fair analogy to suggest that exploring this territory involves embarking on a type of journey, and in order to facilitate this journey I shall first outline the route. I shall start by considering multi-professionalism and team decision making in relation to best practice, and then go on to consider some important theoretical models. This leads to an assessment of the roles and responsibilities of key participants in the exercise, specifically within the domain of English law. En route are encountered issues relating to capacity and consent and the determination of best interests. 'Crunch-time' comes when I discuss the need for a viable framework for critical decision making, and what this might include. The reason it is crunch-time is because here I explain why I avoid relying on the model defined by reference to four 'classic' ethical principles, namely justice, beneficence, non-maleficence and autonomy (i.e. the familiar but limiting 'principlelist' approach to bioethical decision making). The destination is not so much an end-point as an analysis of some key areas that require further research and debate, during which a proposed framework for critical decision making will be first described and then illustrated by means of a case scenario.

# PART 1

# Multi-professionalism and team decision making

The extent to which multi-professionalism is a practical reality depends on the setting within which decisions are made. There is no reason why multi-profes- sionalism should be afforded equal importance in all of the different specialty areas of medicine. The desirability of multi-professionalism as an approach to critical decision making is clear, in that potentially each member of the team has something different to contribute, and according to the Higher Education Funding Council for England (HEFCE) the reason for encouraging multi-profes- sionalism in medical training is 'so that doctors, nurses and other health profes- sionals can work more effectively together'.[1] Theoretically, a multi-professional team ought to be capable of reaching a balanced decision and to benefit from the synergy arising from interaction between various members of the team. However, according to my own research, not everyone believes in the benefits of team decision making, including some more independent-minded clinicians.[2]

It has to be remembered that practical and/or conceptual limitations exist in relation to all models of reasoning. In this chapter I try to argue a position rather than attempting to review differing opinions about the various limitations. The position endorsed is based on acceptance of the balance of probabilities being in favour of multi-professionalism, while acknowledging that acceptance should not be blind to difficulties encountered in the process of translation from theory to practice.

Specialist clinicians are generally trained to think in a particular way, and the evidence base used in their decision making may be particular to their specialty. Accepting that clinical evidence derived from areas such as histology, magnetic imaging and haematology, for example, routinely influences clinical recommen- dations, medical evidence does not normally concern itself with broader patient concerns. Although the need for empirical evidence relating to each patient and each clinical condition is not disputed, this does not preclude the need for additional information in order to provide a more complete profile for each patient. It is not just the diverse nature of information provided that is potentially valuable, but also the nature and quality of interaction between members of a team. Furthermore, interaction ought to extend to include family members, who often have a major role to play, thus helping to inform decisions made by the multi-professional team.

It is to be expected that teams are likely to arrive at decisions via routes that differ from those taken by individuals who are working alone, and not only is there a clinical case for pooling expertise, but also the process has a measure of ethical validity in helping to counterbalance personal judgements formulated from a narrow base of evidence. Such judgements can easily be coloured by different forms of personal prejudice which, apart from anything else, can include favoured clinical treatments that serve the needs of the clinician more than the needs of the patient.

# Theoretical models of decision making

When teaching medical law and ethics, I am often called upon to answer the charge that the subject is imprecise and that there ought to be a right or wrong answer to a given question. That ought to be the case in the context of sitting an examination, but not in the context of a discussion about matrices for critical decision making, and it would be harbouring an illusion to suppose that there were definitively right or wrong answers to all ethical questions. 'Most appropriate' or 'least worst' are more commonly used terms than 'right' or 'wrong' in ethical deliberations. The challenge lies in trying first to identify and then to evaluate the non-clinical characteristics of a proposed course of action. It matters greatly how processes of reasoning are defined if one is to avoid infinite regress, with one question always leading to another, which is a charge that bioethicists can have difficulty in defending. Scientists and medics may feel ill-equipped to 'do philosophy', and some philosophy might be thought to be somehow 'unscientific'. However, this analysis may well be flawed and, historically, functioning in a dual role of scientist/philosopher (or philosopher/scientist) was considered neither impossible nor unusual – consider the examples of Aristotle, da Vinci, Newton, Locke, Darwin and Popper, to name but a few.

*Logical analysis* is relevant in the multi-professional team setting as well as in the context of the deliberations of individual clinicians, and at an informal level, this method of analysis may reliably inform much critical reasoning. Logical analysis can take different forms (e.g. inductive and deductive) and, in broad terms, it can imbue analytic philosophy with a kind of 'internal rigour'. In logical and ethical analysis the processes of reasoning assume a particular importance and are capable of being developed into a whole system of argumentation. Argumentation is a chain of reasoning whereby it is not so much the outcome of a decision that matters as the method and process by which it came about, which typically applies in cases involving complex ethical analysis.

I shall turn my attention next to *justice and democracy* as providing a possible basis for reaching collective decisions. Primarily, the extent to which democratic justice provides a workable model for decision making in the clinical arena is influenced by the hierarchical structures that tend to exist within medicine. Although these may be less conspicuous than they were a quarter of a century ago, when medical decision making was more autocratic and inherently paternalistic, there are issues that remain before principles of democracy can readily find their way into the hospital. Such principles imply a fundamental respect for notions of accountability and justice, which are to be valued. However, what remains contentious, is whether and how principles of justice and democracy apply in a clinical setting.

It is perhaps puzzling that many values associated with modern liberal democracies are founded on notions for which no meta-theory can provide an accurate, comprehensive account, including democracy itself.[3] However, while principles of democracy and justice are unlikely to provide an effective clinical model, partly on account of internal and unresolved complexities, they are indicative of a step in the direction away from medical paternalism.

While majority voting is subject to differences in interpretation and analysis by different political scientists,[3] it is unwise to dismiss the principle too hastily. Collective decision making does not necessarily imply that parties to a decision have an equal voice. Head counting is a crude method to use for formulating clinical decisions, as has long been known. If the number of participants is small, it is mathematically unreliable for trying to reach a just democratic decision.[4] Rather, I suggest that in the medical model equal voting is less important than active participation in the decision making process and demonstrating respect for differences in personal values and beliefs. In the clinical environment, respect for individuals is a significantly more valuable concept than equality of representation.

In terms of mathematical models of decision making, Bayes' rule works on the basis of trying to 'maximize expectations of utility'.[5] In essence, *Bayes' theorem*, which dates back to the early eighteenth century, offers a mathematical formula for calculating probability.[6] It is still used when assessing elements of risk,[7] although it is more likely to be utilised by biostatisticians and epidemiologists than by clinicians, especially in the evaluation of a conceptual (rather than scientific) type decision. While there is certainly evidence of a close correlation between mathematics and philosophy, it has been said that 'the use of Bayes' formula can help to overcome various biases in estimating probabilities such as the bias due to availability, representativeness, anchoring and adjustment, and value-indicated bias'.[7] However, these are broad claims, and Bayesian theory does not offer the most promising method of analysis when it comes to applied clinical ethics, largely because of limitations associated with adopting such a formulaic approach.[8]

I shall now turn my attention to *game theory* in order to consider whether and how its methodology can be employed in the clinical setting. By way of explanation, it has been said that game theory is the most important and useful tool in the analyst's kit whenever they confront situations in which one agent's rational decision making depends on their expectations about what one or more other agents will do, and the decision making of those other agents similarly depends on expectations about them.[9]

However, while game theory pertains to the interaction between different parties to a decision, in the clinical setting two limitations apply. First, there is no provision for key players being unable to participate in the process and it cannot readily be applied to non-competent patients. Secondly, it is unclear whether game theory is able to portray patient–doctor interactions accurately, unless that relationship is characterised by a degree of speculation and mistrust (i.e. malfunctioning).

For example, a patient might answer a question in such a way as to second-guess what the response might be from a clinician, modifying the answer in order to try to achieve a desired personal outcome or goal, which may be completely divorced from so-called clinical need. This is different from exercising personal autonomy – it is about employing a strategy in which key players (in this case the patient and the doctor) modify their behaviour so as to avoid confronting an unwanted fact or eliciting an unsatisfactory response. Such games may well be played out at the bedside or in the consulting room, but that does not give them ethical validity, and it certainly does not mean that they should be upheld as a model for critical decision making.

Game theory concerns the psychology of human behaviour in the social setting, and it can provide a reasonable model for planning strategy. It may be of help in facilitating a team decision, but it is unlikely that patients will cherish the thought of engaging in intellectual recreation, even though it is something that, surreptitiously, some patients may choose to play. Games and numbers are not favoured options in relation to models of ethical decision making, and, to quote from the *Medical Journal of Australia*:

> *Decision making is not truly 'rational' (and is ethically doubtful) when numerical variables are considered to the exclusion of all others ... We need to develop a little 'science of the individual' that can weight all the human and medical factors at play, together with a calculus for clinical judgment that guides the parties to a decision most likely to optimize the chosen outcomes.*[10]

This analysis is helpful and constructive, but I shall revisit the question of risk and calculus in Part 2 of this chapter.

# Analytic jurisprudence

I have arrived at a point where I want to consider some characteristics of jurisprudential models of reasoning. First, to define the term – I use 'jurisprudence' to mean a type of formal analysis about the content and philosophical basis of law, separate from the body of law and its methods of implementation. It is normative in that it reflects the way that law is practised in society, but above all it is a body of knowledge based on moral reasoning and scientific enquiry into the relationship between law and morality. In terms of how it would be employed in the present context, I offer the following hypothesis.

- A theoretical model is needed that can be successfully implemented in a practical setting such as applied clinical ethics.
- Jurisprudence that is ethically sound is broadly based and capable of implementation in a variety of social settings.
- Jurisprudence is ideal for use as an analytic/conceptual tool for critical decision making.

This needs to be carefully argued.

Since Bentham wrote *An Introduction to the Principles of Morals and Legislation* in 1789, much literature has been published on the subject of analytic jurisprudence. The basis of the relationship between law and morals, consciously or otherwise, influences the nature of the discourse between lawyers, philosophers, law makers and practising clinicians. Although healthcare does not feature in their explanations, among others, Austin, Hart, Feinberg, Raz and Coleman,[11] have each provided an informative account of positivist thinking in relation to how law functions in society.

According to legal positivism, law and morals are permitted but not required to have a causal relationship with one another, but there is considerable disagreement about how this relationship can best be explained. One can argue that law and morals are simply different expressions of the same thing, and that it is logically inconsistent to argue that law is based upon anything other than common sense morality, or that moral standards can be defined only in relation to what is or is not lawful. However, these arguments make a number of assumptions about the nature of law, and they fail to capture the essence of the relationship between law and morality, especially aspects of law relating to social interaction (social choice theory or the evolution of the social contract fall outside the scope of this chapter).

The relative interdependence between the twin concepts of law and morality is full of subtleties, not all of which are easy to address. I argue that if one is to avoid deferring to absolute moral principles, and avoid both the assumption that for something to be law it will necessarily also be moral, and the assumption that for something to be moral it will also necessarily be legal, one needs to try to arrive at a fair and reasonable socially inclusive premise. By this I mean that by being broadly based, a set of rules that is conceptually clear and devoid of wrongful discrimination can potentially encourage social inclusiveness and cohesion. As an ethical position it encourages natural social diversity, and encouraging inclusivity as a philosophical position should not preclude practical applications such as occur in the clinical setting.

As a branch of moral philosophy, jurisprudence is capable of scientific modes of application without compromising its ability to help to form evaluative judgements. I maintain that it can defend itself against the charge that it is too abstract with as much ease as it can defend itself against the charge of being too formulaic. It is neither. It can be sharp and analytical and at the same time it can be utilised in such a way that it is entirely sensitive to social and moral concerns. Accepting the limitation that jurisprudence itself is not easy to define, it may be the method of choice when it comes to informing critical decision making and addressing the difficulties of trying to resolve a potentially intractable dilemma. In the next section I shall try to bridge the gap between the theoretical models and their modes of practical application, and to consider how jurisprudential analysis can assist critical decision making.

# PART 2

# Roles and responsibilities

At present, English law is quite specific about who is allowed to decide what and for whom, and in the case of a non-competent adult no one is allowed to consent on his or her behalf. Clinicians alone have to decide on appropriate action that is likely to be in the best interests of the non-competent patient. Scottish law has a system that represents a modification of the North American model, allowing for the appointment of a health proxy, which allows someone nominated by the patient to act as spokesperson and hold power of attorney with regard to medical decisions. Ethically speaking, this is a step in the right direction, and it shows greater respect for people and for the rights of the individual than current English law.

It has to be remembered that however incapacitated a patient might be, that patient remains a person up to and including the moment of death and should be treated accordingly with due respect. I do not believe that this is always currently the case, and I would welcome the chance to redefine the boundaries for decision making and acting in someone's best interests. It is entirely circular to describe such interests by reference to a concept that is so open to interpretation. It presupposes that what is best for one person is probably best for another person similarly placed, which is a rash assumption to make.[12] In the case of non-competent patients, the advice given to the clinician should extend beyond best medical interests, but allowing for the fact that clinicians often have little direct knowledge of a patient, without consultation with someone who knows the patient all that is left for the clinician to do is to second-guess the patient, or to employ a form of substituted judgement, and decide what he or she would want done should the situation be reversed (whereby the clinician was in the role of the patient).

Families may not know what the express wishes of the family member might have been prior to losing capacity, and there may be disagreement within the family about the true nature of those wishes, but some attempt should be made to bring family members into the process of reaching a decision. There are limits to the scope of personal autonomy. Nonetheless, commensurate limits should be set with regards to the deprivation of rights experienced by patients unfortunate enough to have suffered an accident or illness of sufficient seriousness as to deprive them, temporarily or permanently, of the ability to make reasoned judgements for themselves.

# Developing a new framework for critical decision making

Most clinical models for discussing ethical dilemmas defer to the four 'classic' bioethical principles of autonomy, beneficence, non-maleficence and justice (*see* Chapter 1). Although this system has the merit of being familiar, there are limits to its usefulness, not least because of reliance upon abstract concepts that do not sit well with scientifically derived clinical evidence. Such concepts have a tendency to give rise to questions that lead to further questions, or else to defer to absolute moral principles about which there is little or no agreement. The four principles provide a basic taxonomy of ethical categories, but I contend that they are of limited value in the context of applied medical ethics and critical decision making.

It was originally intended that 'the four principles' would provide benchmark reference points for use when assessing the merits and demerits of cases that presented clinicians, patients and patients' families with an ethical dilemma.[13] However, the reality is that these points are not points at all, but broad categories presenting in the form of abstract moral principles. Individual components of a clinical case coming together and presenting parties to a decision with an ethical dilemma are firstly unlikely to sit neatly within a single category, and secondly, if different components pertain to different categories, they can easily be in conflict one with another and hence of little use in trying to find a practical solution. It is one thing for an ethics committee to debate the relative merits of a particular case and to help identify key issues. It is quite a different matter for the clinical team to resolve a problem with the minimum of resources, often under severe time constraints. It is not surprising that clinicians sometimes express frustration at the whole process of ethical deliberation, and there is a clear need for something more workable that has real practical value.

A framework for critical decision making may help to satisfy this need, and I shall outline here one that is currently at a stage of research and development. The framework is meant to expand upon existing recommended legal procedures for seeking patients' consent. At present there are four types of consent forms in ordinary use within the National Health Service to cover the legal formalities that are likely to be encountered in different clinical situations.[14] Normally when the likely outcomes of an intervention are discussed it is on the basis of what a clinician thinks is most likely to happen based on their personal knowledge and experience of similar cases. However, this neither alerts the patient to possible best and worst outcome scenarios, nor does it necessarily present such alternatives as may exist in a way that can be readily comprehended by a non-expert (i.e. such as applies in at least 99% of clinical cases). It should be possible to interview patients and/or their families in a way that can help to guide everyone through the ethical (and not just the legal) process. The interview process should include the transfer of information, and comprehension of relevant information as well as the evaluation of patient comprehension, before a real-life decision is finally made.

The four stages of the proposed framework are as follows.[14]

- **Stage 1 (patient interview).** Take time to ascertain the values system of the patient in question and record key information in the notes. This helps to ensure that when treatment is given it is in accord with the wishes and intentions of the patient. The interview, which is best conducted by the physician in charge or by a senior member of the clinical team, follows a pathway that is to be formatted as a semi-structured interview. In the case of non-competent patients, a similar procedure should take place, but involving a spouse, next of kin or family member closest to the patient. If applicable, an advance directive would be referred to at this point.
- **Stage 2 (review of options).** Define the context of the critical decision in both clinical and resource-based terms to improve the transparency of the decision making process and help put patients (and/or patients' families) in the picture in terms of the available options.
- **Stage 3 (risks and benefits).** Consider the possible or likely outcomes for each intervention or proposed course of action, defining a 'best-practice' ethical standard, as opposed to the basic minimum standard required in law. This stage includes careful evaluation of known risks and benefits, and the charting of these in the notes. The competent patient should play an active part in this discussion unless they insist on delegating this part of the process back to the clinician. Although stage 3 can and should be followed through with non-competent patients, the protocol for involving others is similar to that described for stage 1, while recognising that in England and Wales as yet there is no legal basis for anyone other than the clinician to exercise powers of decision making.
- **Stage 4 (verification and validity).** Present these findings to the patient and/or the patient's family and discuss them with the clinical team. Involving the patient, members of the clinical team and members of the patient's family should help to safeguard against clinical decisions that fail to address non-clinical criteria concerning the patient, and thus reduce the potential for conflict. The use of such methods should be particularly helpful in trying to

avoid treating non-competent patients as if they were non-persons, which is I believe an ever-present risk.

Although it is too early to be able to evaluate the framework, I designed it for use within the hospital setting where difficult decisions have to be made. It may be especially useful where there is little time to reflect, and either there is no clear indication as to the most appropriate course of action or there is disagreement about what this course of action might be. Meaningful communication and exchange of ideas may reduce the likelihood of blame being apportioned in the event of a clinical outcome being unfavourable. This can potentially help to reduce litigation costs for service providers[15] and the wastage of resources that occurs when clinicians spend time in court and in preparation of their legal defence.

The enhanced consent process may help to protect patients and patients' families from avoidable harm, while at the same time helping to promote maximum openness and transparency in the decision making process. The framework is not designed to offer a 'quick fix', but it is hoped that when tested at the bedside it will prove to have benefits, and that it will go some way towards remedying the ethical deficit that tends to occur in the context of a legalistic approach to consent. In the case of non-competent patients where consent is not an option, within the constraints of existing legal protocols the framework should help to protect the rights of patients who are unable to help themselves. It is worth remembering that that person (the patient) could be anyone, including oneself, and when a crisis situation does arise it is too late to begin arguing about protocols or patients' rights. Ethical checks and balances need to be in place first.

# Questions of equilibrium, and discussion points

From an ethical standpoint an attempt should be made to move towards establishing equilibrium within the processes of deliberation. Here by 'equilibrium' I mean 'that state whereby internal forces are in balance, one with another'. This may help to guard against a power imbalance that distorts values attaching to different points of view, and may also help to avoid extremes of viewpoint that militate against reaching a balanced rational decision. However, as a hypothetical position this may not fit within the broader premise of applied ethics, due to making insufficient allowance for personal values, the articulation of which could upset equilibrium and militate against the likelihood of achieving conflict resolution in cases where there is disagreement. If all forces are in perfect balance, which is a true equilibrium, then it might make it more rather than less difficult for parties to the decision making process to identify and agree upon a particular intervention.[16]

In searching for a workable solution to questions about protocol and models of decision making, there needs to be a measure of adaptation in order to facilitate the translation from theory to practice. Even the most refined model for decision making may be insufficiently patient-centred to be of use in the hospital setting, especially if that model lacks flexibility. What is needed is a different type of equilibrium in which all players stand to derive some benefit – not least, of course, the patient. Identifying the desired goal may be a case of balancing hearts and minds, in so far as unbridled rationality can produce brilliant if unworkable hypotheses, and unbridled emotion can cloud judgement about what may or may not be the right thing to do, neither of which is ethically desirable.

Equilibrium has been said to include 'every pair of positive claims that add up to 100%',[16] and in terms of risks and benefits, an intervention that carries a 60% chance of one outcome and a 40% chance of another outcome could be in a state of Nash equilibrium.[17] However, a realistic and acceptable balance is difficult to strike in cases with high levels of unpredictability, in which a significant number of factors remain unknown. This means that if any form of calculus is adopted as part of stage 3 in the clinical framework, it has to be multi-dimensional to be of practical value in the process of evaluation. Probability, likelihood and degree of risk are not synonymous with one another, and it would be wrong to try to oversimplify the assessment of risks and benefits (i.e. by fixing a point on a straight linear scale).

To illustrate how the framework could be applied, consider the following hypothetical case example. In the case of an 80-year-old woman who is dangerously ill in intensive care and suffering frequent lapses of consciousness, enjoying almost no quality of life, a physician might be tempted to conclude that this patient will not want much intervention. In such a case, a 'Do Not Attempt Resuscitation' (DNAR) order might be put on the patient's notes by the responsible medical officer without necessarily consulting anyone else. The patient is non-competent and unable to speak for herself, so under English law the senior clinician has to make a 'best-interests' determination. However, it is clear that this is far from an exact science, and unfounded assumptions can be particularly dangerous to an unconscious patient. In such a situation, the patient's next of kin might want to think that everything possible is being done to save the patient's life, and the question arises as to whether in this case a DNAR accurately reflects the wishes of the patient herself. The clinician may underestimate her physical strength and psychological ability to make a reasonable recovery. Such an estimation could be quite wrong in relation to what is considered 'reasonable', because for one patient being alive may be sufficient in itself, and worthy of sacrifice in terms of pain and suffering, should they regain adequate levels of consciousness. However, for another patient the desire not to endure any further suffering might override all other considerations, and substantial impairments to quality of life could be completely contrary to their wishes, perhaps stemming from a fear of losing independence.

There is evidence to suggest that assumptions made by clinicians in this type of case are often wrong,[18] and the new decision making framework could be beneficially applied. Stage 1 would involve a full and frank discussion with the next of kin in an attempt to try to ascertain what the patient's wishes might have been prior to loss of capacity. If anything had been put in writing (i.e. some form of living will), this would be the time to decide whether or not previously expressed wishes apply to the current situation. If not, then an immediate family member, spouse or partner may well be in a better position to estimate the patient's life-values and choices than a clinician, whose viewpoint is essentially based on clinically related judgment.

Stage 2 would apply if, for example, there was a beds crisis in the hospital, if the patient needed to be transferred to another facility, or if an acute situation arose at the end of a shift, when a clinical team was about to change over. Although routine procedures should be sufficient to cover this type of situation, a decision could well be postponed until the next ward round or until a key member of the team came back on duty. This is perhaps a case of pragmatism rather than advanced ethics, but it is disingenuous to ignore the fact that material considerations can and do apply to the time and manner of decision making.

Stage 3 takes in all of the available information, and factors in the data collected from stages 1 and 2. Risk–benefit analysis is undertaken in the light of specific information relating to an individual patient and the set of material circumstances. By explicitly including these data, when the clinician talks to family members about what happens next (which if possible ought to take place, even though there is no legal obligation to hold this discussion), the information exchange is as meaningful as possible and a considered judgement can be made.

In practical terms the four stages may well merge, and essentially it will be in stage 4 that the critical decision is made (i.e. whether and how to treat). In the case of our octogenarian in intensive care, it might be a question of whether or not to perform cardiopulmonary resuscitation (CPR) if she stops breathing. The possible benefits of a life-saving intervention have to be weighed against either loss of life or a continued life that is only temporarily extended, and which is characterised by severe constraints. If saving life means committing a patient to life support for an indeterminate amount of time, this may not accord with the outcome of stage 1 in terms of that patient's values. Thus, performing CPR may or may not be in the best interests of the patient, and the process is therefore ethically compromised if decision making does not allow for such factors to be part of the deliberations.

When calculating risks and benefits, a number of tendencies are potentially present and pulling in opposite directions. For example:

- risks of serious harm vs. the likelihood of achieving a desirable outcome
- patient values in direct competition with the recommendations of the clinician in charge
- uncertainty about the choice of intervention or course of action on the part of a patient or a patient's family vs. the near certainty that doing nothing will result in further harm or the inability to lead a 'normal' life
- religious orthodoxy indicating the appropriateness or inappropriateness of a particular course of action vs. clinical judgement and independent personal wishes
- wishes of the next of kin vs. the wishes of other members of the family
- an advance directive that is applicable to a given situation, but that is contrary to everyone's intuitions
- cultural values held by the patient and the patient's family that differ markedly from those held by the clinician.

It would be naive to suppose that with so much potential for conflict there is going to be an easy route to follow, or one that will guarantee a good outcome or right answer, however these may be described. Yet the effort has to be worth making, and the purpose of this exercise is to try to identify the method that is most likely to avoid or resolve conflicts, and to come as near as possible to satisfying the implicit demands behind such competing criteria. If the suggested framework succeeds in satisfying ethical requirements without compromising the ability of the clinician to perform a difficult task, then all well and good. If not, it will be for others to try to reach a better solution.

In conclusion, anyone who considers that obtaining consent or making critical decisions on behalf of other people is not especially taxing could be right on occasions. However, such a person could regret not having pondered more deeply when confronted with a case displaying difficult characteristics, such as could well occur in the context of palliative care. If the explanations offered in this chapter help to clarify the consent process, and offer some patients a greater degree of protection, then the effort will not have been wasted. Central to the entire process is the respect that needs to be shown for the rights and needs of the patient – and employing the proposed framework is designed to be a visible and practical demonstration of that respect. It is fair to suppose that, while as yet unproven, some benefits could accrue to all those involved in the decision making process.

# References

1  Higher Education Funding Council for England (HEFCE) press release, 30 March 2001.
2  Worthington R (2003) *Research Project on Capacity and Consent: developing an ethical framework for clinical decision-making.* Funded by the Department of Health, London.
3  *See* Shapiro I (1999) *Democratic Justice.* Yale University Press, New Haven, CT.
4  *See* de Condorcet, Marquis (1785) *Essay on the Application of Analysis to the Probability of Decisions Reached by a Majority of Votes.*
5  *Cambridge Dictionary of Philosophy* (2e) (1999). Cambridge University Press, Cambridge.
6  *See* Gustafson DH, Sainfort S *et al.* (2003) Developing and testing a model to predict outcomes of organizational change. *Health Serv Res.* **38**: 751–76.
7  *See* Hunink M and Glasziou P (eds) (2001) *Decision Making in Health and Medicine.* Cambridge University Press, Cambridge.
8  *See* Kaplan M (1996) *Decision Theory as Philosophy.* Cambridge University Press, Cambridge.
9  Ross D (2002) In EN Zalta (ed.) *Game Theory. The Stanford Encyclopaedia of Philosophy*; http://plato.stanford.edu/archives/spr2002/entries/game-theory/ (accessed 22/3/03).
10  Cox K (2003) Daniel's message for doctors. *Med J Aust.* **178**: 510–11.
11  Coleman JL (2001) *The Practice of Principle.* Oxford University Press, Oxford.
12  *See* Worthington R (2002) Clinical issues on consent: some philosophical concerns. *J Med Ethics.* **28**: 377–80.
13  *See* Beauchamp T and Childress J (1979) *Biomedical Ethics.* Oxford University Press, Oxford.
14  Department of Health; www.doh.gov.uk/consent.
15  Rosenthal M and Schlesinger M (2002) Not afraid to blame: the neglected role of blame attribution in medical consumerism and some important implications for health policy. *Millbank Q.* **80**: 41–95.

16 Skyrms B (1996) *Evolution of the Social Contract.* Cambridge University Press, Cambridge.

17 *See* Nash J (1950) The bargaining problem. *Econometrica.* **18**: 155–62.

18 *See* Curtis RJ, Rubenfeld GD and Gordon D (2001) *Managing Death in the ICU.* Oxford University Press, Oxford.

# 3 Curing and caring

## David Jeffrey

## Introduction

A study of the ethical dilemmas encountered in the course of a serious life threatening illness reveals a tension between concepts of caring and curing. Although palliative care is not limited to any one diagnostic group, it may be helpful to consider the patient with cancer as a paradigm for this ethical analysis of issues surrounding caring and curing.

A diagnosis of cancer may be perceived by a patient as a sentence of death. It is not simply a premature death, but the likelihood of an undignified, painful process of dying, which may frighten the patient. Once cancer is diagnosed, the world becomes unpredictable. People generally have a need to be in control, and uncertainty is difficult to bear. Furthermore, in ordinary language 'cancer' is commonly used as a metaphor for evil. As long as cancer continues to be an 'invincible predator' which is 'obscene' and 'repugnant', then it is likely that patients will be devastated by knowledge of their diagnosis.[1]

The care of a patient with cancer may be divided into phases, each determined by the primary aim of treatment – curative, palliative or terminal.[2]

Palliative care is defined by the World Health Organization in the following terms:

*The active total care of patients whose disease is not responsive to curative treatment. Control of pain, of other symptoms and of psychological, social and spiritual problems is paramount. The goal of palliative care is achievement of the best quality of life for patients and their families. Many aspects of palliative care are also applicable earlier in the course of the illness in conjunction with anticancer treatment. Palliative care neither hastens nor postpones death, provides relief from pain and other distressing symptoms, integrates the psychological and spiritual aspects of care, and offers a support system to help the family cope during the patient's illness and in bereavement.*[3]

Palliative care is concerned with care and communication, whereas mainstream medicine places more value on technology and active intervention.[4,5] These authors suggest that the integration of palliative care into medical care may have blurred the boundaries of care.

# Curing

In the curative phase of treatment there is a realistic chance of cure or long-lasting remission. The aim of treatment is survival of the patient. Some harmful side-effects of treatment may be acceptable to the patient if there is a good chance of cure.[2]

At the time of Hippocrates, holistic health and cure were thought to result from spiritual well-being. The purpose of medicine was not to identify localised lesions, but to explain illness in terms of the total mental and physical disposition of the patient. Caring was an integral part of curing. The linking of the term 'cure' to medical treatment developed in the seventeenth and eighteenth centuries, when hospitals became centres of curing rather than of caring. Cure became interpreted as the removal of physical disease. Medicine became concerned with specific anatomical lesions which could be linked to the symptoms of disease. In the nineteenth century, with the development of technical nursing, hospitals became even more focused on curing, and caring was regarded as a less important activity. The division of cure and care has tended to focus medical attention on removing physical disease rather than exploring the broader notion of the subjective aspects of illness.[6]

The introduction of anaesthesia, modern surgery and antibiotics increased the doctor's potential to cure disease. The scientific advances in cancer care in the twentieth century have encouraged oncologists, radiotherapists and cancer surgeons to adopt a biological view of cancer. Cancer may then be perceived as an organ dysfunction rather than as an illness which affects the whole person. In the quest for the certainty of clinical cure, doctors risk failing to understand the meaning of cancer for the patient. The patient's perception of cure is related to his illness, as a return to the normality which existed before the diagnosis, whereas the doctor's perception of cure is centred on the disease, in terms of five-year survival.

Although historically cure has not been a concept that patients have associated with cancer, with earlier diagnosis and an advancing medical technology, patients with cancer and their families may now have high expectations of modern medicine's power to cure. Such expectations may be fuelled by media reports of 'breakthroughs' in cancer treatment, by medical optimism or by a cultural fear of death.

An advanced medical technology has given doctors the potential not only to cure certain cancers, but also to prolong the process of dying. For instance, the encouraging results of curative treatments for some types of leukaemia have led to the use of chemotherapy regimes for patients with solid tumours such as bowel cancers, where results have been less encouraging. At first such technology was applied indiscriminately to extend life even in those cases where the underlying disease was incurable.[7] Such practices were then considered inappropriate by professionals, patients, their families and the public. Thus a tension currently exists between the availability of life-prolonging treatments with significant side-effects, and a desire to resist the use of such therapies if the quality of life of the patient cannot be maintained.

Nowadays, doctors may be concerned with applying a sophisticated technology to remove disease – the medical concept of cure. Success tends to be measured in years of survival, not in terms of quality of life or freedom from sequelae of cancer. In treatment of a cancer a 'tumour response' may or may not be translated into a survival advantage or better control of symptoms.[2] Iatrogenic side-effects and illness implications may linger for months or years after a person experiences cancer treatment which has been medically defined as curative.[8] In a study of 20 individuals who were pronounced cured, researchers found an enduring sense of vulnerability and evidence that reminders of their illness lingered.[9] Failure to cure in the context of cancer presents particular difficulties for patients facing the unknown, and for professionals who feel that they may have let the patient down.[10]

A dilemma for professionals, patients and patient's families is deciding when to continue to strive to prolong life, and when to focus care on the quality of life and cease active therapies – the dilemma of care vs. cure.[11]

# Caring

'Care' may be defined as serious attention and thought – a person taking caution not to damage or lose, protecting, taking charge of and supervising. The earliest use of the word dates back to the twelfth century, when it was used to indicate 'someone who cared put themselves in a balanced state of mind, providing for the individual, the emotion of sharing with the other their predicament and therefore easing the burden of the person being cared for'.[13] Caring can be caring about someone or caring for someone, or it may imply looking after someone.[14]

It involves the capacity to feel for another person and the capacity to understand something of their situation. In the healthcare context it requires not only an openness to the patient's needs, but also a readiness to reflect on the way that the professionals make judgements about what is best for the patient. Care is facilitative rather than intrusive, and is certainly not invasive.[15]

Caring is thus a physical, social and moral activity. Care is mostly provided by a family in the patient's home. With the demise of extended families and the dominance of the nuclear family, there is less capacity for society to care for the sick at home.[16] Nowadays, care tends to take place in hospitals, hospices and nursing homes, and therefore dying at home is becoming increasingly rare. Care is also provided by the medical, nursing and allied health professionals who make up the multi-disciplinary team.

Much of the literature on caring in a health context is based on nursing practice. Doctors have followed the traditional medical model of care, based on a duty of beneficence. This requires the doctor to do his best for the patient, and also that he causes no harm to come to them as a result of his treatment (non-maleficence). A conflict may exist between a doctor's duty of beneficence – to do what is best for his patient – and his duty to respect the patient's autonomy. This duty to respect the autonomy of the patient is further complicated by a family-orientated approach to care.

Philosophers offer a variety of definitions of autonomy, each focusing on certain facets of this elusive concept. Gillon stresses rationality and liberty in his definition: 'autonomy is the capacity to think, decide and act on the basis of such thought and decision, freely and independently'.[17] In expressing autonomy, an individual shapes and gives meaning to his life. In a situation where death is (or is thought to be) imminent, respect for the patient's autonomy assumes a particular importance. For example, a doctor who believes that a course of chemotherapy would benefit a patient with advanced cancer by extending his life for a few weeks may be tempted not to disclose the poor prognosis to the patient, for fear that he might reject the treatment. By withholding this information the doctor is acting paternalistically.

'Paternalism involves the interference with a patient's autonomy which is justified by referring exclusively to the welfare, good, happiness, needs, interests or values of the person being coerced'. Paternalism is a denial of autonomy, and a substitution of an individual's judgements or action for the patient's own good.[18]

It has been argued that a holistic approach to care is a form of paternalism. The holistic approach may increase patient expectations, and tends to make the patient dependent upon health carers.[19] Such arguments ignore a central characteristic of caring, namely the sharing of mutual respect for the autonomy of both patient and professionals. Thus caring rejects paternalism and works towards shared realistic goals.

The process of dying can be a period of moral development for both patient and professional. Classical philosophical thinking on virtue offers insights into the essential moral nature of caring. Virtue ethics addresses the question 'What sort of person should I be?' rather than the question 'What sorts of action should I take?'[20]

In adopting a caring approach, a member of the healthcare team may develop their moral awareness and hence their moral character and professional maturity. Professional morality and wisdom are developed in the process of confronting ethical dilemmas. These dilemmas may have no 'right' answer, yet they demand a decision.

Ethics is not solely concerned with abstract arguments, but also with the practicalities of supporting patients who may be distressed. Sharing may involve both the doctor and the patient acknowledging their own vulnerability and limitations. Such a close moral relationship requires trust, compassion and the involvement of doctor, nurse and patient. Inequalities of power may act to prevent patients from expressing their views. Sharing involves listening to patients. A partnership between doctor, nurse and patient acknowledges the differences in power but also recognises that all individuals have equal moral status.

# Palliative care

In general, doctors and nurses are more comfortable when treating patients if the goal is cure. In palliative care, the aim is to maximise the patient's quality of life. The transition from a curative to a palliative approach may be filled with uncertainty. The doctor or nurse may feel, or even say 'There is nothing more I can do'.[21]

In contrast to curative treatment, emphasis is placed on the caring aspects of the palliative phase. It is the scientific approach to cure which provides a stark contrast to palliative care, where care is concerned as much with the subjective feelings of the patient and the impact of the illness on the social, emotional and spiritual aspects of his or her life as with the physical disease.

Ashby's risk–benefit analysis model implies that treatment side-effects in palliative care should be less harmful than the effects of cancer itself.[2] Palliative care involves much more than the control of distressing symptoms. It aims to relieve suffering, a more subtle concept which extends to the way in which illness, rather than a disease, affects the whole individual. 'Palliation' was first used in a medical context in the sixteenth century to describe the alleviation of suffering. Palliative care acknowledges the involvement and distress of patient, family, nurse and doctor.[22] For doctors and nurses to deny emotions and feelings of vulnerability in themselves and in their patients is to deny compassion, and to distance themselves from patients.[23] Compassion is an essential part of the nurse–doctor–patient relationship.

In the palliative phase there is a shift in emphasis from quantity of life to quality of life.[24] This shift has an important consequence, namely a requirement to listen to the patient's views. The recognition of the existence of a natural dying process is central to the ethics and practice of palliative care.

Palliative care demands a multi-disciplinary approach rather than a medical one. It is a complex concept which incorporates, yet should be distinguished from, the following: a palliative approach to treatment, which is part of good medical practice; the utilisation of palliative treatments, which includes techniques such as defunctioning ostomies, debulking surgery, orthopaedic fixation and paracentesis. Any of these may be applied at earlier stages of the disease without necessarily adopting holistic palliative care.

Specialist palliative care is a body of knowledge, skills and training programmes which defines the activity of particular doctors and nurses.[25]

Palliative medicine may be defined as the study and management of patients with active, progressive, far-advanced disease for whom the prognosis is limited and the focus of care is the quality of life. The specialty of palliative medicine is thus defined in terms of the stage of disease progress rather than in terms of any particular pathology, body system or technical approach to management,[26] although by using the term 'active', conditions such as dementia and stroke are excluded. The term 'progressive' implies the need for an accurate baseline diagnosis. However, this definition seems to exclude those patients who may benefit from short-term referral to palliative care services early in the course of their disease. Cancer is described as advanced when in someone's clinical judgement it is no longer reversible.[27]

Palliative care is provided when curative treatment is impossible or inappropriate.[28] It may include curative treatment of secondary conditions where this improves quality of life (e.g. antibiotics to treat a chest infection). Similarly, palliative therapies may be appropriate at an early stage of the disease, when the main aim of treatment is cure. It seems illogical to leave patients in pain or distress while they are receiving active anti-cancer therapy, and only to deal with these symptoms at a later stage when they are recognised as 'palliative'.[29] Any distressing symptom that is ignored early in the illness trajectory may be more difficult to control in the last stages of the illness.

There appears to be a difference between palliative care and palliative medicine.[30] This perhaps reflects a perception that medicine is the art or science of the prevention or cure of disease. It involves an active 'doing' based on scientific knowledge, whereas care is offering professional solicitude for another person and implies a more passive process of 'being'. Caring acknowledges patients' suffering, legitimises the experience and gives people a feeling of personal integrity and value.[31] The fact that both of these terms are used within palliative care suggests an uncertainty about the concept of palliative care within the discipline itself. If those who work in the specialty have difficulty in identifying the underpinning philosophy, how much harder this will be for those outside.[30]

Much of the philosophy and knowledge of palliative care was developed within the hospice movement. Hospice care is flexible, individualised, supportive care, including palliative care when appropriate, provided in a hospice, which aims to achieve the best quality of life for the patient and their family and continues into bereavement for as long as necessary.[32] The establishment of hospice care represents a compromise between the over-enthusiastic application of technology to prolong life and the realisation that most dying people do not wish to endure the personal indignities that these technologies may involve.[33]

The greatest confusion appears to relate not so much to the need for palliation but to the timing of it in the spectrum of care.[34] An acceptable definition is needed for several reasons. There may be resentment among other specialists that palliative care specialists are taking over when all that is needed is the palliative approach. In addition, general practitioners need a clear idea of what exactly is being offered to their patients by palliative care specialists.[35] Patients and their families also need to know what the term means, so that they have a clear idea of the goals of care and the resources available to support them.[36] If the patient's disease seems to be resistant to attempts at cure, a clear concept of palliative care may give the professional carers permission to address these issues while curative treatment is still being attempted.[30] In attempting to acknowledge the patient as a person first, the palliative care worker is exposed to the stresses of resolving ethical dilemmas and dealing with his or her own pain and grief. A smooth transition between the curative, palliative and terminal phases of care is facilitated by facing the issues of death and dying. Death-denying attitudes with unrealistic expectations of medicine among both patients and doctors are sources of distress for patients with incurable cancer.[2]

# The transition from cure to palliative care

In the cancer context, clinicians offer differing definitions of the starting point of palliative care. Calman states that palliative care begins when the diagnosis of cancer is established, death is certain and likely in the near future, and a curative approach to care has been abandoned.[37] This statement does not help us in deciding when to abandon a curative approach. It also seems to exclude situations where 'aggressive' chemotherapy is given with apparent curative intent to patients with widespread cancer. Although at a rational level a situation may be clearly palliative, the patient and physician may unconsciously push a goal approaching 'cure' rather than acknowledge palliation. It is possible that the reverse may occur (e.g. when patients with some forms of metastatic cancer are not treated with chemotherapy, when prolonged remission may be achievable).[38] A tension exists between a tendency to 'over-treat' and 'over-investigate', and a fear of 'neglecting' the patient.[39]

Chemotherapy is often given with palliative intent. It is therefore important to assess the effect of chemotherapy on quality of life, and whether it actually does relieve symptoms (i.e. whether it is palliative). There is a widespread tendency to underestimate the toxicity of treatment.[40] Chemotherapy is sometimes used as a way of 'offering hope' in an otherwise 'desperate situation'.[41] However, since this form of treatment carries such a risk of toxicity and does little to meet the patient's real needs for honest, sensitive communication, it should not be used merely to raise false hopes.

Predicting when death is going to occur may be difficult. Specialist palliative care nurses and hospice units emphasise the importance of early referral of patients if the highest standards of care are to be achieved. On the other hand, general practitioners are often faced with uncertainty about the rate of progress of the disease, and defer referral to such specialists until 'the end'.[35]

It is often difficult to know when to switch to palliative care. It may be hard for doctors to acknowledge that they are unable to do any more, and they may have feelings of anxiety and guilt. Honest communication is essential if patients, their families and doctors are to share common aims of treatment. If there has been deception from the start, then doctors will find it more difficult to inform the patient that a cure is no longer possible. Patients or relatives who have drawn doctors into colluding with them may exert pressure to continue inappropriate treatment aimed at cure.[42] Inappropriate treatments may cause harm in a number of ways. Physical suffering may result from the side-effects of such treatment (e.g. hair loss and vomiting from chemotherapy). Distress may also be caused by raising false hopes in the patient and their family. Such inappropriate treatment encourages patients, relatives and doctors to avoid the reality of death. Instead, time should be spent helping the patient to come to terms with his or her death and to address 'unfinished business'. On a wider scale, the inappropriate use of expensive treatments is wasteful of limited medical resources which might have been used to benefit other patients.[43]

# Decision making at the boundaries of palliative care

We need to have a clearer idea of which treatments are curative, palliative or experimental in each clinical setting.[2] George and Jennings suggest that clinical decision making is more difficult when it is certain that the patient will die despite our best efforts.[44] However, it may be that greater uncertainty exists at an earlier stage of disease, when clinicians may be caught in a dilemma between over-treating patients on the one hand, or neglecting some remote chance of cure on the other. In palliative care, health may be perceived as an ability to conclude life appropriately and to derive meaning from that living until death.[30] Patients may be suffering an unresolved past, unsatisfactory present and a lost future. There is often a blurring between acute and palliative care. George and Jennings suggest that we are going to have to become problem solving and perspective solving with regard to our patient, thus balancing buying time with buying quality. The legitimacy of buying time may be reasonable. There is a need to explain the costs of going down the curative side, in terms of unfinished business, tasks, relationships and personal resolution. Because the boundaries of care are blurred, it may be more appropriate to shift our attention to respect for the patient's autonomy. George and Jennings make a distinction between 'acute palliative' and 'palliative palliative', and suggest that we should aim to break down the barriers between cure and palliative care.[44]

The failure of chemotherapy, radiotherapy or surgery to cure advanced cancer may cause palliative care physicians to neglect the use of these approaches when they may be helpful.[30] Conversely, oncologists may feel that palliative care is easing a patient into an earlier death than is necessary. Sadly, a state of two solitudes may exist where the two fail to consult each other adequately. Palliative care physicians must be familiar with advances in oncology. There is a need to integrate palliative care at an earlier stage in the disease trajectory. Furthermore, there is recent evidence that general practitioners and primary healthcare teams are uneasy and feel a sense of guilt about the quality of care that they are providing for patients with incurable cancer at home.[35,45] Difficulties in professional relationships can raise fears among general practitioners that specialists may take over the care of patients.[46] Hospital care on the other hand may not offer a suitable environment for the process of dying.[29] Slevin has shown that oncologists vary enormously in their choice of treatment for advanced cancers.[47] Mackillop *et al.* have also shown that although the patient, doctor and family may share a common understanding initially, as time passes and the cancer progresses, patients and physicians may develop divergent views about the aims of the therapy. Patients in a palliative setting may well believe that therapy is aimed at disease control.[48]

It may be appropriate to identify the uncertainties that exist at the boundaries of palliative care and to clarify the issues involved. The uncertainties involve the patient and their carers.

# Uncertainties at the boundaries of palliative care

## Uncertainties for doctors

There is a risk that doctors may lose sight of a cancer's potential to cause death. For instance, in widespread metastatic disease there is a dilemma. To what extent should we spend resources hunting for the primary tumour? Estimating the prognosis for an individual patient is notoriously hazardous. How much of this uncertainty should be shared with the patient? Clinical uncertainty is such that there may be a very real possibility of buying good-quality time for someone who may appear moribund, either with aggressive interventions or by adopting judicious palliative measures. Who should make the decision to switch from curative to palliative care? Palliative care demands a team approach to care. To what extent should the patient be included in decision making? Reaching a moral consensus within a multi-disciplinary team may be difficult.

Nowadays, a conflict often exists between technical care and personal care. In the context of modern medicine, time to listen to patients may be perceived as a luxury.[49] Medical training concentrates on clinical competence, and there is a danger that compassion may become a redundant value. Ethical dilemmas represent one of the most challenging aspects of medical care. Struggling with questions which have no obvious answer is an essential part of the professional role.

In striving to act with integrity, honesty and a sense of moral responsibility, we define what lies at the heart of what it means to be a professional.

## Uncertainties for nurses

Much of palliative care is nursing care. Traditionally nurses are closer to patients and more aware than doctors of the wider needs of the patient. These needs, which may be psychological, social or spiritual, may be of greater significance to the patient than his or her medical problem. Nurses may be placed in a situation where they have to act as an advocate for the patient. They may then be faced with loyalties divided between patient, doctor and manager. Advocacy is a useful mechanism for power sharing within the team, but all too often it is perceived in a negative way – as a threat, or an implied criticism of medical care. Doctors need to listen to their nursing colleagues, who often have a broader view of the patient's concerns. It is illogical to treat patients as equals, but not colleagues who happen to work in a different discipline.

Nurses may also feel uncertain if there is no clear team philosophy. A patient with advanced cancer may ask a nurse how serious his condition is. How is the nurse to respond if she knows that the consultant always gives an optimistic prognosis?

## Uncertainties for patients

Calman defines quality of life in terms of the gap between a person's expectations and the reality of his or her situation.[37] Where there is a wide discrepancy between expectation and reality, quality of life is low. Calman's model serves to emphasise that part of a doctor's role may be to help patients to have more realistic expectations, particularly at the point where the focus of care is changing from curative to palliative.

Palliative care aims to maximise patient autonomy, so long as it does not adversely affect the autonomy of others.[21] Taking responsibility for his choices may mean that the patient will blame himself if events turn out badly. At the interface between curative and palliative care it is particularly important to give patients their final opportunity to exercise their autonomy. Patients are tougher than we think. Part of the task facing the professional carers is to make some evaluation of the quality of the patient's life. It is important to remember that the most reliable assessor is the patient him- or herself.

Quality of life relates both to objective features of disease and to subjective feelings, hopes and fears. The concept of quality of life extends beyond a balance between the impact of a treatment and its side-effects to recognise and respect the autonomous individual – the patient in the social context of their relationships with family and friends.

Patients need just as much information to make rational decisions about their medical condition as they do for any other sphere of their lives. If the doctor is uncertain at the transition from curative to palliative care, he needs to acknowledge his vulnerability and seek to share his concerns with his team, which includes the patient.

## Uncertainties for relatives

There may be a feeling of helplessness and a perception that their loved one is suffering. Relatives often fear the harm that might be caused by giving honest information to the patient. They may insist that the doctor must not tell the patient that cure is no longer possible ('The news would kill him, doctor'). This is how collusion is born. As it develops it isolates the patient from their loved ones, their doctor and the nursing staff.

Respect for the patient's autonomy demands that at least they should be the first to know what is happening. This may be difficult if the patient is still drowsy following surgery, or if cerebral function is decreased or compromised for some other reason. Professionals can help by suggesting that relatives are present at these discussions.

The relatives may insist that 'something must be done'. Doctors need to explain that palliative care does not mean giving up care. Relatives are often unfamiliar with the features of the normal dying process.

# Palliative to terminal care

During the terminal phase of illness all unnecessary treatments are withdrawn and 'no treatment-related side-effects are acceptable'.[2]

The phase of terminal care involves the last days of a person's life, when death with dignity is the aim of care. Relatives may express their distress in terms such as 'I would not let a dog suffer like this.' This may surprise the professional carers, who see a patient who seems to them to be dying peacefully. Carers may also become distressed if dying seems to be prolonged. Perhaps patients die as they have lived – some with quiet acceptance, others 'raging at the dying of the light.'[50] We have duties of care to ease suffering, but not to hasten or prolong the process of dying. In the past, people used to die at home in familiar surroundings, whereas now there is an increasing trend towards death in hospitals. Dying with dignity means different things to different people. We need to distinguish between euthanasia, palliative sedation, control of pain and withholding or withdrawing life-prolonging treatments.

Euthanasia is the deliberate termination of a person's life. Palliative sedation is the intentional administration of sedative drugs in the dosages and combinations required to reduce the consciousness of a terminal patient as much as is necessary to adequately relieve one or more refractory symptoms.[51,52] The control of pain has nothing to do with euthanasia, since its purpose is to relieve pain, not to end a life. Withdrawal of treatment in the course of illness occurs when the time arrives when it is no longer possible to restore health, functions or consciousness, and it is no longer possible to reverse the dying process. At this stage, the most that even the most aggressive therapy can achieve is to prolong the dying process.

Patients are not obliged to undergo treatment that is futile and physicians are not obliged to begin or to continue such treatments.[53,54] Doctors need to accept that death is a part of life. Death may come as a relief, but it is not an option for doctors as a means of achieving relief.[44]

However, doctors may be placed in a difficult situation by relatives who equate continuing active treatment with maintaining the patient's hope and morale.[6] These attitudes are one consequence of the medicalisation of death. Death is no longer a familiar natural event. Dying is often perceived to be a frightening, painful process which should occur in hospital rather than at home.

# Multi-disciplinary teamwork

Patients with cancer often present a wide range of physical and emotional problems which can threaten to overwhelm the individual doctor or nurse. A team of professional carers from different disciplines that share the aims of palliative care can have the strength and skills to meet the various needs of the patient. However, working in multi-disciplinary teams can lead to inter-professional rivalries, leadership difficulties and delayed decision making, and may generate unrealistic patient expectations.[55] Thus ethical problems of inter-professional power sharing can have a detrimental effect on patient care.

Successive National Health Service (NHS) reorganisations have not made multi-disciplinary working any easier. However, professionals do need to define their areas of expertise so that each understands the other's potential contribution to care. Specialist nurses whose skills are not recognised may become demoralised and deskilled if they are not allowed to make an appropriate contribution.

No individual member of the team should be seen as less significant than another in a team partnership.

As professionals we need to acknowledge the moral challenge of seeing the patient as a whole person by sharing access to the patient. The sad alternative is to witness the prospect of doctors and nurses directing care so as to maintain their inter-professional boundaries, to the neglect of the patient and their family. Respecting the autonomy of fellow professionals in different disciplines breaks down inter-professional boundaries and creates a team spirit that is directed towards achieving the aims of palliative care.

The vital 'care' component of nursing work is difficult to identify and measure. It is this 'caring' element which is vulnerable in an organisation that is driven by economy and efficiency. Such market forces operating within the NHS have threatened the provision of the 'invisible' components of holistic care of dying patients.[56] Nurses want to work as part of a team, supporting each other and accepting individual responsibility for their decisions. If doctors and nurse managers do not respect the autonomy of nurses, these nurses will be unable to offer the highest standards of care to their patients. Sharing information within a team is a mechanism for sharing power and respecting the autonomy of other team members.

If members of a team respect the autonomy both of the patient and of fellow professionals, then they need to share power and be willing to accept responsibility for their own decisions. To develop such a sharing relationship is to form a partnership – not just between professional carers but also including the patient.

General practitioners, district nurses, hospital consultants, ward sisters and other healthcare professionals are equal partners and need to recognise each others' skills and roles if they are to meet the needs of patients. Professionals from different disciplines need to communicate and negotiate the optimal plan of care with the patient and their family. This partnership preserves respect for the autonomy of both patients and professionals by a process of joint decision making and goal setting.[57] Partnership depends upon trust and an acceptance of the patient's view as valid and important. In an everyday work situation, such trust involves a recognition of the uncertain nature of palliative care in the community. Trust involves supporting the intuitive clinical skills of the team, skills which can only flourish in a secure, safe environment. Expectations of other team members should be realistic, and their contribution needs to be acknowledged. A trusting environment allows for open, honest discussion of views, which in turn promotes further mutual trust. This type of partnership, underpinned by the ethical principles of respect for autonomy, challenges paternalism or individualised leadership by the doctor. As mentioned earlier, it seems illogical to treat patients as equals, yet to treat one's colleagues as inferiors merely because they may work in another discipline or be employees.

# Models of care

Ethical frameworks based solely on abstract theories of deontology or utilitarianism may seem difficult to apply in a clinical situation. Utilitarianism may seem to discriminate against the individual cancer patient, while the impersonal duties of deontological theory may be inappropriate for the emotional aspects of the care of a patient who is suffering. Both of these theories attach great weight to pure reasoning and appear to reject and mistrust emotions. They also seem to ignore the practical effects of the difference in power between professionals and their patients.

Similarly, models based on the quartet of autonomy, beneficence, non-maleficence and justice are most useful in abstract analysis, but less helpful in the setting of close relationships.[58,59] If an ethical framework is to be of practical use to patients and staff, respect for autonomy needs to be combined with a caring approach. Such a model has the advantage of acknowledging that feelings, compassions, integrity and virtue play a vital part in the holistic approach to care.

Ethical decisions need to be considered in the context of an individual clinical case and not just in abstract isolation. It is the doctor rather than the nurse who makes the decision to change from a curative to a palliative approach. This decision legitimises the patient's entry into the dying process.[56] Field distinguishes between 'clinical death' (the absence of life signs such as respiration and heart beat) and 'social death' (the process whereby staff, relatives and friends withdraw from the terminally ill). Open, honest communication between staff and patients creates a relaxed atmosphere. In this setting, the mutual respect, trust and friendliness between doctors and nurses can lead to their skills being used in an optimal way.[56]

A patient-oriented approach concentrates on the need for full information and sets limits on the doctor's perception and beliefs. In his willingness to inform, a doctor reveals his respect for the patient's autonomy.

The central function of informed consent is to ensure that there is a sharing of power and knowledge between doctor and patient. Through this sharing process the patient receives appropriate care from doctors whom they trust, and doctors gain a deeper understanding of the patient's needs.

Informed consent can be viewed as an expression of two elements of care – one responsive to the patient's wishes and the other protective against harmful intervention.[60] Informed consent is a dialogue between a patient and their doctor in which both become aware of the potential harms and benefits for the patient. Thus informed consent is much more than a mere granting of permission.

There is a need for a better understanding of decision making under conditions of uncertainty at the boundaries of palliative care. Doctors may have a notion of what it is to be 'scientific', namely that if the causes of an illness are unclear, more tests must be performed. However, a conflict exists between this objective attitude and an empathetic approach. We need a model of decision making which combines a requirement for scientific rigour and technical competence with an ethical duty of compassion and respect for the patient's autonomy. We need objective scientific knowledge, but we also need wisdom.

For doctors and patients to face uncertainty together there has to be trust between them. We cannot make wise decisions when we deny the existence of uncertainty. Acknowledgment of uncertainty removes a barrier to trust, gives a sense of control over the outcome, and offers doctors and patients a chance to be allies rather than adversaries. Thus by giving up the illusion of total certainty and sharing the reality of uncertainty, we can make more realistic decisions. It is only when we face the fact that we are taking chances that we can begin to make choices. If patients and their families are involved, the doctors gain the benefit of their knowledge and the support that comes from sharing the diagnostic and therapeutic dilemmas which previously the doctor had borne alone. Thus more flexible decision-making strategies, together with a consideration of a wider range of possible causes, lead to better decisions and better care, and to increased trust between doctor and patient. Our minds get used to thinking in terms of whatever tools we use. If we only have a hammer, then every problem looks like a nail. Scientific decision making in curative care can be contrasted with a consensus team approach involving the patient in palliative and terminal care.

George and Jennings have devised a model of decision making that is based on respect for patient autonomy.[44] Applying a therapeutic index or balancing cost benefit may be expressed visually as a beam, balancing curative (pathology-based) and palliative (symptom-based) options on a fulcrum that represents the patient's agenda.

Patients need time for doctors and nurses to listen to their views. Treatment of the cancer may have ceased, but care of the patient continues until the moment of death.

| Curative | Patient agenda | Palliative |
|----------|----------------|------------|

| | | |
|----------|----------------|------------|
| **Pathology** | **Fulcrum** | **Symptoms** |
| Diagnosis | Tasks | Wasted time |
| Curability | Relationships | Side-effects |
| Prognosis | Unfinished business | Complications |
| Buying time | | Polypharmacy |
| | | Buying quality |

Society needs to reach an agreement about the proper care of the dying. It is possible that many individuals would be able to die at home, with their families around them, and without the use of expensive 'high technology', if they were well informed and allowed to choose the place in which they were going to die.

## A caring model[21]

A partnership between healthcare professionals and the patient involves:

- a commitment to teamwork
- a holistic approach to care
- acknowledging uncertainty and vulnerability
- listening to the patient
- avoiding distancing.

Promoting acceptance of death and resolving unfinished business involves:

- demystifying cancer and death
- acknowledging the value of life and rejecting euthanasia
- accepting that 'letting the patient die' may be permissible
- making an appropriate transition between a curative and a palliative approach to care, with the patient's consent and comprehension
- taking account of the patient's view of quality of life.

Caring for the carers involves:

- supporting the patient's family
- supporting doctors and nurses.

The key to coping with the various uncertainties which arise when beginning and ending palliative care lies in the process of sharing. Doctors need to share their uncertainty with patients and their families and with their nursing colleagues. Informed consent is a mechanism for sharing the power of doctors and the patient.

# Conclusions

Rapid advances in cancer treatments and the search for cures have created a division between scientific technical care and personalised palliative care. These differing approaches have evolved their own philosophies of care, resulting in the creation of a boundary between curative and palliative care. Palliative care has changed over the past 30 years to become a more scientifically rigorous discipline. Perhaps it is now appropriate for those who adopt technological curative strategies to assimilate some of the holistic approaches of palliative care. Care is different from active treatment whose results can be quantified. Care respects the dignity of the patient and acknowledges his or her humanity.[5]

If healthcare professionals work together with the patient and their family in a true partnership of care, respecting autonomy and seeking informed and understood consent, then we shall have a better chance of achieving our therapeutic aims – whether they are curative or palliative.

# References

1 Sontag S (1979) *Illness as Metaphor*. Penguin, Harmondsworth.
2 Ashby M and Stofell B (1991) Therapeutic ratio and defined phases: proposal of an ethical framework for palliative care. *BMJ*. **302**: 1322–44.
3 World Health Organization (1990) *Cancer Pain Relief and Palliative Care. Technical Report Series*. World Health Organization, Geneva.
4 ten Have H and Janssens R (2002) Futility, limits and palliative care. In: H ten Have and D Clark (eds) *The Ethics of Palliative Care: European perspectives*. Open University Press, Buckingham.
5 ten Have H and Clark D (eds) (2002) *The Ethics of Palliative Care: European perspectives*. Open University Press, Buckingham.
6 Faithfull S (1994) The concept of cure in cancer care. *Eur J Cancer Care*. **3**: 12–17.
7 Brody B (1988) *Life and Death Decision Making*. Oxford University Press, New York.
8 Loescher LJ *et al.* (1989) Surviving adult cancers. Part 1. Physiologic effects. *Ann Intern Med*. **111**: 411–32.

9  Shanfield S (1980) On surviving cancer: psychological considerations. *Comp Psychiatry*. **21**: 128–34.

10 Hurny C (1994) Palliative care in high-tech medicine: defining the point of no return. *Support Care Cancer*. **2**: 3–4.

11 Brody B (1988) *Life and Death Decision Making*. Oxford University Press, New York.

12 Hawkins JM (ed.) (1986) *The Oxford Reference Dictionary, New Illustrated*. Clarendon Press, Oxford.

13 Eyles M (1995) Uncovering the knowledge of care. *Br J Theatre Nurs*. **9**: 22.

14 Brown JM, Kitson AL and McKnight TJ (1992) *Challenges in Caring*. Chapman Hall, London.

15 Barker P (1989) Reflections on the philosophy of caring in mental health. *Int J Nurs Stud*. **26**: 135.

16 Gracia D (2002) Palliative care and the historical background. In: H ten Have and D Clark (eds) *The Ethics of Palliative Care: European perspectives*. Open University Press, Buckingham.

17 Gillon R (1985) *Philosophical Medical Ethics*. John Wiley & Sons, London.

18 Dworkin D (1972) Paternalism. *Monist*. **56**: 64–84.

19 Girad M (1988) Technical expertise as an ethical form: towards an ethic of distance. *J Med Ethics*. **14**: 25–30.

20 Hursthouse R (1999) *On Virtue Ethics*. Oxford University Press, Oxford.

21 Jeffrey D (1993) *There is Nothing More I Can Do: an introduction to the ethics of palliative care*. Patten Press, Penzance.

22 Cherny NI, Coyle C and Foley KM (1994) Suffering in the advanced cancer patient: a definition and taxonomy. *J Palliat Care*. **10**: 57–70.

23 Alderson P (1991) Abstract bioethics ignore human emotions. *Bull Med Ethics*. **May**: 13–21.

24 George RJD (1991) Palliation in Aids: where do we draw the line? *Genitourin Med*. **67**: 85–6.

25 Thorpe G (1993) Palliative care comes of age. *Hosp Update*. **2**: 435–6.

26 Doyle D, Hanks G and MacDonald N (eds) (1993) *The Oxford Textbook of Palliative Medicine*. Oxford University Press, Oxford.

27 Cassem EH (1985) Appropriate treatment limits in advanced cancer. In: JA Billup (ed.) *Outpatient Management of Advanced Cancer*. Lippincott & Co., Philadelphia, PA.

28 Sutherland R, Hearn J, Baum D and Elston S (1993) Definitions in paediatric palliative care. *Health Trends*. **25**: 148–50.

29 MacDonald N (1995) The interface between palliative medicine and other palliative care services. *Proc R Coll Phys Edinb*. **25**: 558–68.

30 Pennel M and Skevington S (1994) Problems in conceptualizing palliative care. In: R MacLeod and C Jones (eds) *Teaching Palliative Care: issues and implications*. Patten Press, Penzance.

31 Schuman A and Matthews D (1988) What makes the patient–doctor relationship therapeutic? Exploring the connexial dimension. *Ann Intern Med*. **108**: 125–30.

32 Sutherland R, Hearn J, Baum D and Elston S (1993) Definitions in paediatric palliative care. *Health Trends*. **25**: 148–50.

33 Charlton R, Dovey S and Mizushimay Y (1995) Attitudes to death and dying in the UK, New Zealand and Japan. *J Palliat Care*. **11**: 42–7.

34 Doyle D (1993) Introduction. In: D Doyle, G Hanks and N Macdonald (eds) *The Oxford Textbook of Palliative Medicine*. Oxford University Press, Oxford.

35 Jeffrey D (2000) *Cancer: From Cure to Care*. Hochland and Hochland, Manchester.

36 Roy DJ and Rapin C (1994) Regarding euthanasia. *Eur J Palliat Care*. **1**: 57–9.

37 Calman K (1988) Ethical implications of palliative care. In: M Freeman (ed.) *Medicine, Law and Ethics*. Blackwell Publishing, London.

38 Hurny C (1994) Palliative care in high-tec medicine: defining the point of no return. *Support Care Cancer*. **2**: 3–4.

39 Kearsley JH (1989) Compromising between quality and quantity of life. In: BA Stoll (ed.) *Ethical Dilemmas in Cancer Care*. Macmillan, London.

40 Kearsley JH (1986) Cytotoxic chemotherapy for common adult malignancies: 'the emperor's new clothes' revisited. *BMJ*. **302**: 1–2.

41 Brett AS (1988) The patient's expectation in the United States. In: BA Stoll (ed.) *Cost Versus Benefit in Cancer Care*. Macmillan, London.

42 The A-M, Hak T, Koeter G and van der Wal G (2000) Collusion in doctor–patient communication about imminent death: an ethnographic study. *BMJ*. **321**: 137–8.

43 Rees GJ (1991) Cancer treatment: deciding what we can afford. *BMJ*. **302**: 799–800.

44 George RJD and Jennings AL (1993) Palliative care. *Postgrad Med J*. **69**: 429–49.

45 Donald AG (1995) Palliative care in the community: difficulties and dilemmas. *Proc R Coll Phys Edinb*. **25**: 550–7.

46 Royal College of General Practitioners and the Cancer Relief Macmillan Fund (1995) *Palliative Care Facilitator Project*. Royal College of General Practitioners and the Cancer Relief Macmillan Fund, London.

47 Slevin ML (1990) Attitudes to chemotherapy: comparing the views of patients with cancer with those of doctors, nurses and the general public. *BMJ*. **300**: 1458–60.

48 Mackillop WJ, Stewart WE, Ginsberg AD and Stewart SS (1988) Cancer patients' perceptions of their disease and its treatment. *Br J Cancer*. **58**: 355–8.

49 Howie JGR, Heaney DJ, Maxwell M, Walker JJ, Freeman GK and Harbinder R (1999) Quality at general practice consultation: a cross-sectional survey. *BMJ*. **319**: 738–43.

50 Thomas D (1982) 'Do not go gentle into that good night'. In: S Heaney and T Hughes (eds) *The Rattle Bag*. Faber and Faber, London.

51 Brockaert B and Olarte JM (2002) Sedation in palliative care: facts and concepts. In: H ten Have and D Clark (eds) *The Ethics of Palliative Care: European perspectives*. Open University Press, Buckingham.

52 Cassem EH (1985) Appropriate treatment limits in advanced cancer. In: JA Billup (ed.) *Outpatient Management of Advanced Cancer*. Lippincott & Co., Philadelphia, PA.

53 British Medical Association (2000) *Withholding and Withdrawing Life-Prolonging Medical Treatment: guidelines for decision-making* (2e). British Medical Association, London.

54 General Medical Council (2002) *Witholding and Withdrawing Life Prolonging Treatments*. General Medical Council, London.

55 Fottrell E (1990) Multi-disciplinary functioning: will it be of use? *Br J Hosp Med*. **43**: 253.

56 Field D (1989) *Nursing the Dying*. Tavistock & Routledge, London.

57 Wilson-Barnett J (1989) Limited autonomy and partnership: professional relationships in health care. *J Med Ethics*. **15**: 12–16.

58 Gillon R (1985) *Philosophical Medical Ethics*. John Wiley & Sons, London.

59 Beauchamp TL and Childress JE (1983) *Principles of Biomedical Ethics*. Oxford University Press, Oxford.

60 Baum M, Zilkha K and Houghton J (1989) Ethics of clinical research: lessons for the future. *BMJ*. **299**: 251–3.

# 4 Giving it straight: the limits of honesty and deception

## Heather Draper

## Introduction

Hearing that you are going to die sooner than you had thought, or hearing that the best that medicine can offer by way of a cure has not cured you, is for most people, devastating news. We may take out insurance to cover our premature death, but we do not really expect to need it. A terminal diagnosis is perceived by healthcare workers as one of the worst pieces of bad news to have to give – save perhaps that of telling a parent that their child is beyond cure. It is the kind of news that alters the course of someone's life and at a stroke ends all their hopes for the future and many of their perceptions about themselves (e.g. as independent, competent or supporting – rather than supported – members of the family). But of course this news is not always what the patient most dreads, nor need it herald unadulterated gloom. For patients who are weary of a dutiful struggle against a long-standing illness, the opportunity to stop fighting the illness and concentrate on living might be welcome. For others, the news, although undesirable, might come with hitherto unconsidered benefits. Although many of us hope for a sudden and painless death, if we simply never come home from work one day this can be more devastating for our families than coming to terms with a forthcoming death and making plans together for the future up to and beyond the funeral.

Recently, for a close friend of mine, the terrible and unexpected news that her father had only a few more months to live was turned into a tremendous gift, as she and he were reconciled with each other in a way that she had never dreamed would be possible. Both of them would have been robbed of something very precious if he had not been told that he was dying. Moreover, he was able to die in his own home because he was able to discuss openly and honestly his pain relief and other needs with his carers. My friend was able to suspend her studies and return home to help her mother to care for him. His death was distressing for all the family, and I am sure that the intensity with which my friend still misses him has been heightened by their total reconciliation, but the experience was nevertheless a positive one. This is one case where honesty and the best that palliative care could offer turned the bad news into something positive for everyone concerned.

Equally, we have all heard of cases where the news of a pending and premature death heralds the beginning of unremitting misery, hopelessness and defeat. Everyone has had the experience of a patient who 'turned their face to the wall', and it is impossible to ensure that every patient, no matter how angry and resentful they (or their family) are, will have a peaceful death. In the above case, my friend readily admits that she would never have predicted that her father's premature death would have been such a positive experience. In many respects, none of us know how we will respond until we have to so.

In palliative care, being honest with patients about their prognosis has always been considered a first principle. Being referred for palliative care at all generally means that the patient has been told their prognosis, even if they refuse to believe it. Is honesty in palliative care simply a pragmatic requirement, because good palliative care may be frustrated unless the patient is dealt with honestly? The answer is clearly not, for receiving good palliative care is not just a matter of receiving the best that palliative care can offer. It impacts on the quality of life and death, relationships, and present and future interests. The use of the word 'good' in 'good palliative care' (or 'good medicine', or 'good nursing', or 'a good doctor' or 'a good nurse') has two meanings. It is both a technical assessment and a moral judgement, because maximum health is one of the 'goods' of life. It is a good from which other goods flow, and it is also a means to an end of achieving other goods. Because good healthcare has a moral as well as a technical component, and because giving and receiving healthcare involves the formation of relationships, we are likely to ask the same questions about honesty in a therapeutic relationship as we are in any other relationship. Is it obviously the case that in this relationship 'honesty is the best policy'? Should we always 'tell the truth and shame the devil'? We can all think of circumstances where nothing but harm can be caused by an honest reply, but we still hold fast to the belief that honesty is a virtue and deception is to be avoided.

There are three possible responses to this problem. The first is that we should always be honest, and that when we are not, either we are being weak-willed (or cowardly, even) or we are being overly paternalistic. The second response is that deception can indeed be a good thing on occasions, and that what we need to do is to determine when these occasions arise. The third response is that honesty is a character trait that adapts to circumstances, and is not to be interpreted as a statement that one never lies or deceives.

Each of these responses can be explained and justified with reference to the central ethical theories of Kantian deontology, utilitarian consequentialism and virtue ethics, and questions about honesty and deception extend beyond those of giving a terminal prognosis. Overlying all of these problems in the therapeutic relationship is the extent to which the professional is under a greater obligation to be honest with the patient than with others, and whether the duty of care may on occasions require a limited amount of deception – perhaps even a degree of deception that would be unacceptable in non-therapeutic relationships. However, before we move on to look at theories and other examples in the later sections of this chapter, we need to be certain of what it is we mean when we say that we applaud honesty and deplore deceit. Is honesty the same as always telling the truth? Is deception always achieved through lying? These are important questions, for it is not unusual for people to claim that although it is permissible to remain silent, it is impermissible to lie – even though the predicted effect is the same. Likewise, it is commonly asserted that it is one thing to tell the truth, but quite another to tell the whole truth, because being 'economical with the truth' is not the same as lying. Distinctions such as these are controversial, and exploring the potential difference helps to clarify not only the terms we use, but also the importance bestowed.

# Honesty and deception, lying and truth-telling: conceptual differences

Todd and Still[1] surveyed the strategies and tactics of GPs communicating with their terminally ill patients. We would not be surprised to learn that in 1993, many GPs often tried to disclose bad news (as they perceived it) by allowing the patient to dictate the pace at which understanding was reached. What was surprising was that another strategy was to avoid disclosure, using the tactics of evasion, denial, uncertainty, hints and prompts, euphemism and inappropriate reassurance. Here are some of the things that GP 20 said about their means of avoiding the issue.

*I never tell them what they have got ... even if the hospital has told them ...*
*I always try to make them see it differently ... that they didn't understand it*

*... that it is not terminal, it will clear up.... I just don't give it [the terminal diagnosis] away.... I always try to avoid answering ... or I try to be cheerful and change the conversation.... They will ask things like 'Doctor, do you think I will benefit from going to hospital?'. I say 'Yes, you will benefit', even if I do not think that they will.... I may well tell lies like ... 'We have got a letter from the hospital [saying] that they are hoping that you will be all right in the next month or so, but you need to get over the operation' ... [once] I just said that I am sorry that I don't have the full [report of the] investigation from the hospital yet.... I didn't tell this woman anything.... In fact, to get out of it I sent one of my colleagues to go instead of me because I knew that she would put me in a corner ... and that worked because she didn't ask him.... I told him I couldn't tell her that she had cancer.... I don't think he told her anything, she wouldn't have asked him. But I never saw her again.*

It would be seriously unjust to make inferences from the practice of this GP about the practice of healthcare workers generally. What is interesting about this GP is that they employed several different means of avoiding honest communication with the patient – particularly evasion. Although there is admission of direct lying, something akin to the truth is also being used either to evade or to deceive. Imagine a patient asking 'Do you think I have a chance?' and being told 'Well, I sincerely hope so'. It may be the case both that one has this sincere hope, and also that it is very unlikely to be realised. However, the net effect on the patient is likely to be that they do think that it is realistic to hope. In other words, they are as deceived by the truth as they may have been by the straightforward lie 'Yes, I think you have a chance'. Of course, we can also reconcile ourselves to our deceptions by crossing our fingers behind our backs as we speak, thinking 'There is always a chance – no matter how slight, it is still a chance'. We know that we are deceiving, but we feel better about it because we have not lied.

Examples such as this suggest that the real principle at issue here is not truth-telling but honesty. In medicine only one thing seems certain, and this is that our 'knowledge' of 'the truth' is constantly changing. It is not unlikely that most of what we now believe to be the truth will, in the future, be shown to be mistaken belief. In this sense, we may rarely be imparting 'the truth', however well intentioned and committed to honesty we are. We would, however, draw a distinction between mistakenly misleading someone (because we are misinformed) and deceiving someone. It is not truth-telling which is important to us, but honesty.

Jennifer Jackson[2] makes several other useful comments on truth-telling. The first is that, whatever we may claim, we actually lie quite frequently. The examples she gives include signing 'Yours sincerely' or responding 'Very well thank you', when we actually barely know the person whom we are addressing, or we feel dreadful. This behaviour is not quite the same as endorsing so-called 'white lies'. Little white lies tend to be characterised by the relatively trivial nature of the deception involved. The untruths we tell almost as a matter of protocol or etiquette are different in the sense that they are not meant to be believed. They fall outside the parameters of honesty because we all know the rules. We are not deceived, nor is there any intention to deceive. This leads to a second observation, namely that in order to deceive, the deceiver has to be believed. I might tell you the most terrible lie, but if you do not believe me, you are not deceived.

There is a difference between the intention to deceive and the success of that intention. It is not obvious that the failure neutralises the act. Although it may be consequentially better for intentional deception to fail, there is something morally suspect about this intention which exists independently of the outcome. Jackson's third observation is that people deceive without the intention of doing so – for example, because they do not realise the interpretation which has been placed upon their behaviour. However, should they become aware of this deception and fail to correct it, they become party to the deception. It becomes voluntary even though it was not intended. For instance, Nurse Roberts raises his eyebrows to acknowledge the discreet arrival at Ms Ghupta's bedside of a colleague who is late for the ward round. Roberts' gesture coincides with the consultant informing Ms Ghupta that the effects of chemotherapy are really not so bad. Ms Ghupta notices Nurse Roberts' gesture and thinks that it signifies that he disagrees with the consultant's opinion about the chemotherapy. She decides not to consent to the chemotherapy without a second opinion. Nurse Roberts, when talking to her about her decision, realises what has happened, but does not inform Ms Ghupta of her error. Although his original gesture was not intended to misinform Ms Ghupta, he becomes party to her deception when he fails to correct her false impression.

To summarise, it is never possible to be certain that one is telling the truth, because one might be misinformed. However, one can be honest and genuinely misinformed, and this suggests that what counts is not the imparting of the truth *per se*, but the intention to be truthful. It is also possible to deceive someone unintentionally. However, if this unintentional deception is deliberately left unchecked, then one might be considered to have voluntarily deceived, even though there was not any original intention to deceive. Likewise, one can intentionally deceive by deliberately manipulating the truth so as to misinform.

This also suggests that it is honesty rather than truth-telling as such which is important. Similarly, deception requires the person on the receiving end to be deceived, which suggests that the dishonesty of the person intending to deceive can be evaluated independently of the good or bad consequences which flow from the intention.

# Is there an ethical imperative to be honest?

This seems a strange question to ask, because it provokes the response that it is obvious that we should be honest. The problem with this answer is that there are occasions when being honest will do only harm, and in such cases it seems at least permissible, if not required, to be dishonest. It is probably our reluctance to let go of the general principle of veracity that causes us to 'fudge the truth' on those occasions when dire consequences will follow if we are honest. After all, hard cases make bad laws. However, it is also commonly asserted that health-care ethics depend upon four principles – autonomy, non-maleficence, beneficence and justice – and that these principles sometimes conflict with each other, generating the hard cases. Looking to the consequences of our actions – as we must in order to assess their benevolence or maleficence – permits us to be flexible and to recognise that although it is generally benevolent to be honest, it is legitimate to be dishonest on occasions.

This approach would be justified by utilitarianism. Honesty is generally the best policy, because without it we could not depend upon people to be honest. A wholesale erosion of trust would be a sufficiently weighty negative consequence to outweigh some specific benefit of dishonesty or problem with honesty. When I ask for directions or for the correct time, I assume that the answer given will be honest (even if it turns out to be mistaken or unclear, as so many directions are!). A general adherence to honesty is necessary for trust to exist between members of society, particularly relative strangers. However, in other relationships, including those between patients and carers, a more explicit relationship of trust exists. The quality of the care that we experience depends almost as much upon the trust we have in our carers as it does on their skills and competence. Where trust breaks down, so does care. This is a strong utilitarian reason to be honest, but utilitarianism cannot embrace absolute adherence to rules. Where honesty promotes only harm, we are free to abandon it. However, cases where honesty promotes only harm are rare. Generally we have to achieve a balance of harms and benefits, which might mean that dishonesty does do harm, but not as much – or so we hope – as being honest would. The balance of harms and benefits in healthcare recognises that the trust of patients is fragile, and that the benefits generated by dishonesty can be quickly outweighed by the harm of losing a trusting relationship. For instance, if we lie to a patient at the request of a relative, we have to consider not only whether a breakdown of trust with the patient will result (should the lie be discovered), but also whether our willingness to lie will jeopardise future relationships which the relative might form with other practitioners. If one practitioner is willing to lie at the request of a relative, how can that relative be certain that another practitioner will not lie to them if requested to do so? We should also consider that even when the predicted good consequences do flow from lying, the deception always harms people to some extent because it undermines their autonomy.

Utilitarianism does give weight to the effect that lying has on autonomy. Mill, for instance, argued that maintaining autonomy itself has vitally good consequences that should never be taken lightly. In this respect, the principles of non-maleficence and beneficence conflict with the principle of autonomy less frequently than arguments in favour of paternalism often suppose. Doing well for people includes promoting their autonomy, and non-maleficence can concern itself with the protection of autonomy.

Kantian ethics give a different weight to autonomy than does utilitarianism. Mill's argument for permitting maximum liberty was that a society in which the liberty to challenge the status quo is limited is liable to stagnate and crumble, which is in no one's interests. Kant held that autonomy is inextricably linked to morality, and that it is therefore nonsense to be both in favour of morality and willing to undermine autonomy. He argued that it is our capacity to be autonomous which generates ethical duties. This is because in order to be responsible at all we must be capable of exercising our own will, choosing our own ends, and choosing between courses of action (maxims) which will meet those ends. Kant's second formulation of the categorical imperative (test for moral conduct) was that we should respect the autonomy of others by never using autonomous people solely as a means to our own ends, but always treating them as ends in themselves. Being dishonest with someone is an example of treating them as a means to our own ends. For instance, if we lead a patient falsely to believe that his diagnosis is not terminal, because we believe that the bliss of ignorance is better than the pain of knowledge, we deprive him of the opportunity to decide for himself which is of greater value. In addition, we deprive him of other choices which he would be in a position to make if he knew the truth about his condition. In both of these senses, we make him a means to our ends and we fail to respect his autonomy, depriving him through his ignorance of choice, because as a direct result of our deception we prevent him from making critical decisions.

In addition, Kant argued that moral choices were also wholly rational choices and that just as rationality was universal, so too was morality. In this respect his first formulation of the categorical imperative, namely universality (that we should ask how it would be if everyone did what we were proposing to do), also acknowledges the relationship between honesty and trust. If everyone lied all the time (i.e. if lying were universal), the whole purpose of lying would be undermined because no one would ever believe that they were hearing the truth. Accordingly, it is self-defeating to lie, and irrational to act in a self-defeating way.

Kant furnishes us with two reasons for making honesty an absolute rule. His views about the unconditional value of morality and autonomy enable him to assert that telling lies is always wrong because if something is unconditional – without conditions – it admits no exceptions. It is universal. Interestingly, it is at this juncture that Jennifer Jackson defends the distinction between telling lies and intentional deception. She proposes that although lying is always wrong (for the reasons generally attributed to Kant, namely that it is imperative to have an absolute prohibition on lying, in order to maintain trust and autonomy), intentional deception may be benign, and therefore, permissible in circumstances where it would be wrong to lie. Bakhurst[3] disagrees with this view. He argues that since intentional deception and lying amount to the same thing (the patient is denied access to the truth), if lying is wrong (for the reasons given by Jackson) then intentional deception must be equally wrong.

Jackson's response to this claim is to draw a distinction between those cases where intentional deception undermines trust (as lying always does) and those cases where it does not. For instance, both intentionally deceiving a patient and lying to her in order to gain her consent to some treatment are equally wrong. One cannot be absolved of the wrongs of lying by substituting intentional deception, because in both cases the trust that the patient has is undermined (to their detriment in terms of autonomy). However, Jackson claims that a betrayal of trust 'can only occur in those cases where those being deceived can reasonably have expected not to be', and that what we can reasonably expect is culturally determined, not absolute. Although she concedes that the present culture of western medicine is autonomy-centred, she recognises that it need not be so. For instance, it could be driven by an understanding of non-maleficence which is not founded in respect for autonomy. Likewise, by extension, it is possible to envisage that even within our autonomy-centred culture, individual patients might want to base their relationship of trust with their carer not on the promotion of their autonomy, but on the belief that the carer will always act in their best interests as perceived by the carer ('You decide, doctor – I know that you will do what you think is best'). This is a similar, but not identical situation to the one in which patients autonomously let their doctors make the decisions ('You decide, doctor – you're the expert').

If this distinction is valid, it removes one of the stumbling blocks to deception in healthcare (palliative or otherwise), namely that patients need to be told the truth in order to consent to therapy. In a model of healthcare where autonomy is the prominent value, consent is vital as an expression of autonomy, and being informed is vital to consent. However, we need to remember that this is not the only model of healthcare in operation, and that it is as paternalistic to force a patient to conform to this paradigm as it is to prevent them from doing so if they wish.

However, this is an extremely limited defence of deception, and one where dishonesty is related only to the betrayal of a particular kind of trust. It is far more common for defences of dishonesty to be made on the basis that autonomy, although important, is not absolutely important and can be outweighed by other considerations, such as different harms to self (e.g. longevity and well-being), or the erosion of the autonomy of others or the avoiding of different harms to them. These distinctions, and their significance, are best illustrated by reference to the examples which will be discussed in the following section.

The final theory against which to measure the imperative to be honest is virtue theory. Virtue theory has its origins in ancient Greek philosophy, one aim of which was to discover which kind of life is best for humans to live. It is recognised that what counts as a virtue cannot be determined solely by asking questions about what 'good' is or means, because any definition of 'good' is influenced and conditioned by circumstance. For this reason, virtue theory holds that people need to be trained to be good so that they acquire the habit of goodness through practising being good. To be truly virtuous is to know spontaneously what should be done because of the kind of person one is. For this reason, whereas both utilitarianism and Kantian ethics start with the question 'What should I do?', virtue theory asks 'What kind of person should I be?'. If I want to be a good palliative care practitioner, I need to know what qualities good palliative care practitioners have. To learn this, I may look around for a role model to emulate, and by emulating this role model I will acquire virtuous characteristics myself. Virtuous qualities need not be universal, for instance, a good jazz musician will need different qualities to those required for palliative care – but it is likely that some virtues will be common to similar professions.

One criticism of virtue theory is that we need to be able to recognise good practice in order to emulate it, and that we therefore run the risk of perpetuating bad practice. This was the charge levelled against healthcare practitioners some 30 years ago before it was decided – partly due to public pressure and partly due to legal judgements – that practitioners should be encouraged to develop their own skills of ethical judgement. However, virtue theory has been growing in popularity in recent years as the professions have begun to return to the view that being a good practitioner owes a great deal to attitude.

The virtue theory view of honesty enables practitioners to be more responsive to circumstances than deontology allows, without binding them to considering only the consequences of their actions, as utilitarianism does. Possessing the virtue of honesty does not commit us to telling the truth on each and every occasion. The virtuous person knows when it is important to be honest and when to exercise discretion. The mark of the virtuous person is that whatever they do on any one particular occasion, they retain our respect as honourable and upright people whose judgement is trusted.

# Honesty applied

## Being selective with the truth

The advantage of thinking in terms of honesty rather than truth-telling is that we can draw a distinction between bluntness and truthfulness, and between honest and dishonest selective truthfulness. Children often fall foul of these distinctions when they are instructed 'Always tell the truth' and then proceed to do so indiscriminately – just as the word 'always' suggests that they should. Honesty can be legitimately tempered with compassion. It is common practice when communicating with patients to let them dictate the pace at which information is given. Breaking news gradually is not dishonest. The 'whole truth' need not be delivered in an instant, provided that one intends to make oneself available to respond honestly to requests for more information.

Likewise, it is not dishonest to keep unsolicited opinions to ourselves. For instance, it is not dishonest to keep to oneself the opinion that a family should visit more often, or stay for less time, or address different issues on their visits. Likewise, it is not dishonest of me not to offer the view that your shirt is awful and your breath smells. Similarly, one should distinguish between offering professional advice and personal advice when asked during the course of one's work for advice about what someone should do. When we do offer unsolicited information we may be motivated by considerations other than honesty. For instance, informing a family that their visits are too long might be part of the duty of care owed to a patient who becomes exhausted or distressed during extended visits. There is a sense in which we are always selective with the truth. The practice only acquires negative connotations when the selectivity is part of a conscious effort to deceive.

## Confidentiality

Further evidence that we are under no absolute obligation to disclose the truth comes from a consideration of confidentiality. Being truthful or honest is compatible with not disclosing everything we know when we have a duty to maintain confidentiality. The duty of confidentiality attempts to draw a distinction between that which is known and information that, although it is known by someone else, we own and have a legitimate right to keep to ourselves. We can be party to information which is not ours and which we cannot therefore disclose. However, this duty is not an uncontroversial one, particularly when there are concerns that others might be harmed as a result of their ignorance, or when rigid adherence to confidentiality is perceived by relatives as being obstructive or antagonistic.

In recent years, discussions about confidentiality have tended to focus on the dangers of refusing to disclose the positive HIV status of a patient to individuals at risk of infection. However, a dilemma about whether or not to disclose confidential information can be generated by far less dramatic concerns.[4] In palliative care, carers might be asked not to tell relatives about the seriousness of a patient's symptoms or his decision to minimise intervention. However, carers have also been asked not to tell relatives apparently good news, as the following case study illustrates.

## Case study 4.1

Against all the odds, and despite being referred to a hospice, Collette showed signs of recovering from bowel cancer. After several months, the consultant decided that Collette was no longer terminally ill, although he could not be certain that she would not become ill again in the future. Accordingly, he felt that she no longer needed the extensive support supplied by the hospice, and he discharged her. Collette was very upset about this, partly because she did not want to lose her terminally ill status, which had generated rather more attention from her family than she had been accustomed to in the past. The hospice staff were not unsympathetic. They had, after all, promised Collette that they would not abandon her and that they would care for her until she died. There was also a widely shared belief among the staff that Collette's family had rather neglected her in the years preceding her diagnosis. Because they did not wish to let Collette down, she was given a radically reduced but honorary status as an outpatient. For instance, she still attended some social events, and she had her hair set by a hairdresser who donated some of her spare time to the hospice. It quickly became obvious that Collette's family did not realise that she was no longer thought to be terminally ill. The nurse-manager attempted to talk to Collette about this, but was politely and firmly told to mind her own business.

## Discussion

Collette's circumstances are obviously not usual, and her success in keeping her new prognosis from her family was aided by the attempts of the staff to negotiate a new relationship with her. Whatever one thinks about the wisdom of the staff's decision to maintain a relationship with Collette, the principal argument in support of honesty, namely that it enables autonomous decision making, applies to Collette's family, too. It is not unlikely that if they were in possession of all the facts, the family would reduce the company and help they were prepared to give to Collette. Irrespective of how unreasonable their predicted behaviour might seem to either Collette or the staff, neither should prevent the family from making their decision for themselves. However, the staff are obliged to keep Collette's medical history confidential, despite the fact that what they are keeping from the family on this occasion might be classed as good rather than bad news, and despite their judgement that Collette was being at best imprudent, and at worst wrong not to update her family. Clearly, the staff will feel even more awkward about the situation if any members of the family begin to ask direct questions. A further cause for concern is the hairdresser who is volunteering her skills to help people who are terminally ill. Unless she is informed that Collette is no longer terminally ill, she is being deceived into parting with her voluntary labour every time she sets Collette's hair.

One point to be made about this case, and others like it – even when there is more at stake, as in the case of an undisclosed HIV risk – is that autonomy is double-edged. Being responsible for one's decisions – as Collette is asserting that she is – not only gives one the freedom to decide for oneself, but also leaves one open to praise or blame for the decisions one makes.

## Consent and the choice to be ignorant

We have already discussed the distinction between autonomously deciding to let other people make one's therapy decisions, and the type of relationship that is based on a different kind of trust, namely that the carer just does always have one's best interests at heart. Calliope Farsides discusses these kinds of decisions at length in Chapter 6 of this book.

One of the problems with these decisions – like those in Case 6.2 (*see* page 90), where Jean deliberately excluded herself from decisions about her care – arises if the patient has requested that they should not be reminded of their deterioration. Randell and Downie[5] discuss the case of one such patient with breast cancer, in whom metastases in the cervical spine were discovered. This indicated that the patient should take more rest and wear a neck collar to minimise the risk of quadriplegia. In a case such as this, those charged by the patient with her care have to decide whether to talk to the patient about this further deterioration, or to respect her wishes not to have anything discussed with her. If they respect her wishes, she may not realise the full significance of their advice to wear a neck collar. Farsides' case of Dillon in Case 6.1 (*see* page 88) is similar, in that the patient has chosen to be only partially informed about the unscrupulous practices of drug companies.

## 'No good can come of telling them the truth'

There are very few cases where there is nothing to be said in favour of honesty. Usually the erosion of autonomy or the adverse effects of discovery carry some weight, even if they are ultimately thought to be outweighed by the harms that being honest could cause.

## Case study 4.2

Mrs Stretton was under the care of a palliative care consultant in a general care-of-the-elderly ward when she took an unexpected and acute turn for the worse, and died before her family could be with her. The family, as is common in these circumstances, asked about Mrs Stretton's death –

whether she had said anything or suffered. In fact, Mrs Stretton had become very distressed because she realised that she was dying before she had expected to, it had not been possible to keep her pain-free and she had asked where her family was.

In circumstances such as these, it might seem more than permissible to intentionally deceive, or even to lie. Telling her family cannot change Mrs Stretton's experience of death, and they could be plunged into guilt and remorse about something over which they had no control.

However, there are occasions similar to this when even though no good can be generated in the particular circumstances, dishonesty might store up trouble for the future. Suppose that Mrs Stretton had not been told that she was terminally ill, at the explicit request of her family, and that the staff (against their better judgement) had acceded to those wishes, even though they believed that Mrs Stretton's care was being compromised, particularly when she realised that death was imminent. Although one might still be tempted to keep the distress of her death to oneself, greater consideration would need to be given to reassuring her family that they did the right thing in not telling her that she was dying.

We need to draw a distinction in this context between repeatable and unrepeatable occurrences. Clearly, if the event is unrepeatable, the assertion that nothing can be gained and only harm can be done looks valid. However, since it is likely that the family will have to deal with terminal illness on future occasions, it is highly desirable that they learn from their mistakes – however painful this might be at the time.

Palliative care was one of the first specialties to take team or shared care seriously. Honesty plays an important role in building a strong team. Everyone must feel able to voice support or misgivings, to acknowledge their mistakes and triumphs, and to take as well as give without fear or resentment.

However, teamwork also has its problems. It is not clear where the responsibility lies for decisions made by a team. Is it like a democracy where all agree to accept the decision of the majority, or do individual members have a veto? Does the most senior member of the team carry ultimate responsibility, or are all equally and jointly liable for any mistakes that are made? Does one person canvass the opinion of all and form a final judgement based on these views, or does the team have to reach a compromise on which everyone can agree?

Teams that have resolved these and other problems are likely to be well established, with a history of trust and loyalty between members. What would a member of such a team do if she discovered that a colleague had set the filtration on a syringe driver too high, bringing about the premature death of a terminally ill patient? We might like to apply the same repeatable–unrepeatable distinction which was used in the previous example, advising her to speak out only if she believed that her colleague was liable to repeat this mistake.

However, this decision is not without risks. It is not difficult to imagine that the first in anyone's long line of eventually discovered mistakes was perceived at the time to have been a 'one-off'. Likewise, amassing decisive evidence of someone's incompetence is a matter of balancing the effects of a premature claim against the harm that they may inflict during the period when the evidence is amassing.

# Summary

The aim of this chapter was to raise questions about what leads us to commend honesty and to avoid dishonesty. It is impossible to give hard and fast advice about when dishonesty may be justified, if indeed it ever is. It has also been suggested that on at least some occasions when we 'fudge the truth', there is nothing to choose between this and lying, even though our prohibitions against dishonesty are generally phrased in terms of lying, and our commendations of honesty are couched in terms of truth-telling. It is important to recognise that a good deal of dishonesty can be promoted through evasion, silence and even truth-telling. At the same time, it is important to recognise that our obligation to be honest does not extend to giving unsolicited advice or opinions, and neither is honesty always promoted by bluntness. Honesty is not simply about being prepared to disclose the truth – some people are not entitled to it, as all who are bound by a duty of confidentiality know. Allowing patients to accept or take responsibility for their own actions is difficult enough when they are only harming themselves. It is even more difficult when the well-being of others is at stake.

In this chapter the issue of honesty has been addressed almost exclusively as if it were the burden of practitioners. We should not forget, as Farsides (see Chapter 6) also reminds us, that patients are also moral agents with their own moral burdens, honesty included.

One of the tensions of being a professional is generated by the recognition that one's own actions may have adverse consequences for the profession as a whole. Although I agree with the sentiment that honesty is a stable character trait that permits exceptions and discretion, the repercussions of dishonesty may resonate further afield than we anticipate. This is particularly true in palliative care, which has a commendable history of investing considerable effort in treating dying patients openly and honestly.

# References

1 Todd C and Still A (1993) General practitioners' strategies and tactics of communication with the terminally ill. *Fam Pract*. **10**: 268–76.
2 Jackson J (1991) Telling the truth. *J Med Ethics*. **17**: 5–9.
3 Bakhurst D (1992) On lying and deceiving. *J Med Ethics*. **18**: 63–6.
4 Draper H (1997) Confidentiality. *J Med Defence Union*. **13**: 28–30.
5 Randell F and Downie RS (1996) *Palliative Care Ethics: a good companion*. Oxford University Press, Oxford.

# Further reading

Jackson J (1993) On the morality of deception – does method matter? A reply to David Bakhurst. *J Med Ethics*. **19**: 183–7.

# 5 Advocacy and palliative care

## Robert Stanley

**Advocacy** ... I. *The function of an advocate; pleading for or supporting.*[1]

## Introduction

Within palliative care, as in other forms of health and social care, advocacy is commonly understood as speaking up for someone else. In particular it embraces self-advocacy, through which people are given support in their palliative care in order to speak for themselves. It is the process of facilitating their autonomy – however vulnerable, and whatever their level of dependency. It is important that the patient's voice is heard because with consultation, dialogue and co-operation, care is more likely to be effective. Advocacy is a process which involves information gathering, making the information accessible, discussing choices, facilitating decision making by the individual and monitoring outcomes. The palliative care practitioner has an important role in this process, since it involves prognosis and care.

The strengthening of patients' rights through advocacy and empowerment can be summarised as follows.

- Patients should not be treated as objects by healthcare agencies. Even though a patient may have commenced their death, they should be allowed to take their own responsibilities, and supported in this. Patients can only take responsibility and contribute to their own healthcare if they are well informed and respected.
- Healthcare should be aimed at the patient's needs. Humanness and compassion should replace paternalism. To achieve this, patients' rights should be strengthened. More and better information is the first condition that should be met in order to achieve this.

- Patients should be assisted in becoming better informed about the possibilities and quality of available services. This should cover all aspects of cure and care. Structures for disseminating accurate and up-to-date patient information should be strengthened.

Members of the multi-disciplinary palliative care team have a responsibility to protect the patient's interests, even (where necessary) defending those interests against a perceived threat from other members of the team.

For a palliative care service to be truly patient-centred, it must be infused with the views and values of the public (as patients of the past, present or future). The public must be involved. In the present-day context, patients' rights constitute an important aspect of everyday hospital practice. The right to be informed about one's health, the right to take an active part in the process of palliative care, the right to be educated and counselled in managing a life-limiting illness or the commencement of death and coping with everyday life, and the right to have a better quality of life – are all issues that have emerged during patient-oriented activities in recent years.

# Guiding principles

Palliative care is a moral enterprise invested with mutual respect and trust between caregiver and patient. The maintenance of integrity in the professional conduct of care encompasses responsibilities to patients, employers and colleagues. There is a need for democratic values, honesty, courage, diplomacy, and respect for the patient's autonomy.[2]

A range of meanings have been given to the term 'autonomy'. Gerald Dworkin summarises this diversity well:

> ... 'autonomy' is used in an exceedingly broad fashion. It is used sometimes as an equivalent of liberty ... sometimes as an equivalent to self-rule or sovereignty, sometimes as identical with freedom of the will. It is equated with dignity, integrity, individuality, independence, responsibility, and self knowledge. It is identified with qualities of self-assertion, with critical reflection, with freedom from obligation, with absence of external causation, with knowledge of one's own interests.... It is related to actions, to beliefs, to reasons for acting, to rules, to the will of other persons, to thoughts, and to principles. About the only features held constant from one author to another are that autonomy is a feature of persons and that it is a desirable quality to have.[3]

Hill takes a more systematic approach. He distinguishes between distinct, though related forms of autonomy,[4] including the germinal sense in which Kant used it in his *Groundwork on the Metaphysics of Morals* as a property of the will of rational beings to act in accord with principles. Hill also refers to the Sartrean autonomy, to the sense of autonomy as the ideal rational life, and to modern concepts of autonomy as a psychological capacity and a right. A hybrid of Kantian and the latter two concepts informs the more recent bioethical constructions of autonomy by Veatch,[5] Beauchamp and Childress,[6] and Gillon.[7] The influence of bioethical discourse into law has further altered the meaning of autonomy and brought it closer to, if not sometimes synonymous with, doctrine on self-determination.[8] As such it is reduced to a right, principally to refuse treatment, if the criteria for autonomous decision making are satisfied. Generally these are as follows:

- understanding
- belief
- choice.[9]

Seedhouse[10] rejects what he sees as a narrow, conventional view of autonomous decision making. He advances a position on autonomy as an intrinsic quality of people, he espouses creating autonomy and he acknowledges the place of power in enabling autonomy.

It may seem obvious that health professionals should fully inform a patient about their care, discuss the options available and obtain their consent to what is being proposed, because to act otherwise is to disregard the patient as an autonomous being. It is trite now to assert that patients have a right to give their informed consent. However, to say that health professionals should have respect for a person's autonomy has wider implications than this. If it is accepted that an autonomous person, having been presented with the facts, makes a rational decision about the kind of treatment they want, then in order fully to respect that person's autonomy, healthcare practitioners must accept whatever decision the patient makes. This can cause conflict for the practitioner between their concern for the patient's well-being and their respect for whatever decision the patient may make (e.g. when a patient refuses life-saving treatment because of a religious belief, or attempts to commit suicide).

Who counts as a person for the purposes of commanding equitable treatment and respect? John Rawls proposes that 'a person is someone who can be a citizen, that is, a fully cooperating member of society over a complete life,' but adds 'for our purposes . . . I leave aside permanent physical or mental disabilities so severe as to prevent persons from being normal and fully co-operating members of society in the usual sense.[11]

In response to Rawl's conceptualisation, Ruth Anna Putnam asks 'Are we to conclude that a permanently disabled human being is not a person, or at any rate not a citizen?'[12]

From an agency-focused moral perspective, such an individual's status will be relativised to whatever physical, sensory or cognitive performances are designated as crucial expressions of moral activity. The less replete and flexible the repertoire of instrumentally valuable performances, the less inclusive the theory will be in attributing full moral agency to individuals whose powers to perform differ from the normal or customary range.

Critiques of the emphasis on autonomy as a prerequisite for moral agency or of respect for autonomy as the basic moral value have been raised by both communitarians and feminist ethicists. The communitarian critics have claimed that the emphasis on autonomy presupposes an atomistic individualism (i.e. a view of moral agents that sees them as totally separate, and not embedded in social relationships which precede their individuality). Communitarian critics of autonomy point to the deleterious effects of too great an emphasis on respect for autonomy which, in their view, will lead to a collapse of communities and eventually into a state not much different from a Hobbesian state of nature. The feminist critics claim that the emphasis on autonomy flows from a masculine tradition in moral philosophy, and builds on a neglect of the moral experience of women. The feminist critique has much to inform palliative care in that it shares part of the communitarian critique and adds a further set of observations about the importance of the caring relationship for our understanding of the moral life. The masculine emphasis on rights and duties is seen as a truncation of the moral life which must be rectified by a care ethic that gives moral weight to relationships. Within the context of palliative care, such an ethic will focus not on the isolated individual and his or her rights and duties, but on that individual within a set of caring relationships.[13]

A criticism which is commonly levelled by both communitarians and feminists is that self determination constitutes a hopeless and therefore an unfairly imposed goal for people who are powerless and vulnerable, and especially for those who have commenced their death, or who have an incurable illness. They argue that to be inclusive of individuals who are too frail or otherwise compromised to conform to this paradigm, moral theory should promote relationships that bond powerless individuals to more powerful ones. Annette Baier,[14] for example, contends that the inequality manifested in dependence connects caregiver and care recipient morally by exposing them to mutual risk. For the relationship to work, each gives up control because each is, figuratively speaking, a hostage to the other's role. This mutuality of dependence constitutes the paradigmatic moral bond. Those with end-stage or incurable disease who would benefit from care should not lose this autonomy. Immanuel Kant advises any prospective benefactor to 'show that he is himself put under the obligation by the other's acceptance or honoured by it',[15] so as to forebear from placing the recipient of help in an inferior position. Kant's example illustrates how, in the context of reciprocally constraining practice, individuals can be interdependent yet self-determining. Thus interdependence can be accepted as integral to human life. As Kant suggests, drawing individuals of differing power together in a mutually binding moral space is facilitated when, regardless of how needful one is of assistance by the other, social practice maintains reciprocity between them.

Empowerment goes beyond the narrow focus on rationality in the discourse on self-determination and patient autonomy by recognising the person's power. Such empowerment serves to facilitate each person's individual fulfilment, with wider implications than those suggested by rational choice. As Feste notes, 'The empowerment model speaks of self-awareness, personal responsibility, informed choices and quality of life'.[16]

However, the reference to personal responsibility does not abandon the patient to looking after him- or herself alone. An important dimension to empowerment is that it fosters knowledge of and reliance on self in relation to the interdependence of all resouces, human and other. Patient autonomy and self-determination, on the other hand, historically favour individualism and privilege.

The process of self-awareness and the process of taking control are consistent with the notion of self-help, and are indeed often conflated with empowerment. However, empowerment loses its political edge if it is seen only as another form of self-help or enablement.[17] Although the ends of empowerment may share some of the ends of self-help, a radical and vital aspect of empowerment lies in its recognition of the power relationships between healthcare practitioners and patients.[18]

# Protecting rights

Empowerment involves facilitating and encouraging patients to engage in these choices and rights themselves. Much of the literature on empowerment emphasises this at a number of social levels of interaction and action. Athena McLean, while noting the operation of empowerment at an individual level, also identifies three further levels:

1 group – involving self-help and mutual aid
2 organisational – effecting change in the social community
3 consumer – securing greater funding and promoting advocacy.[19]

Action at all of these levels may help to effect patient empowerment with regard to palliative care. The role of healthcare professionals is therefore to provide information, impart knowledge and offer guidance. The main challenge arises from the need to ensure that the palliative care is being patient led and not prescribed, that the decision making is not being disempowered. In addition, there is a professional challenge to engaging in patient-led care, yet still maintaining boundaries, high expectations and realisable outcomes.

The growing body of self-efficacy research provides important insights into how people heal. Even with regard to the process of dying and life-limiting illness, the process of empowerment lies at the heart of healing. The key to empowerment is to offer tools, skills, information and support for self-help.

Dr Dean Ornish, President of San Francisco's Preventative Medicine Institute and a leading researcher on the effects of lifestyle on heart disease, makes the following comments:

> *The notion of empowerment is critical because there's a lot that's pretty disempowering about modern medicine. But physicians who behave in a way that undercuts patients' sense of self-efficacy may actually have a negative effect on their health.*
>
> *I think that even more than feeling healthy, people want to feel free. That is why I don't believe in doctor's orders. If I order patients to do something, I'm not really empowering them. I may even be making the problem worse. My goal is to help people gain power and freedom. Because only then can they become more responsible.*
>
> *One of the most empowering things physicians can do is to help people understand how their problems are related to their lifestyle and thinking. The idea here is not to blame them or make them feel guilty, but to provide an opportunity to take responsibility. Illness can become a catalyst for getting people's attention, and starting them on the path to empowerment.*[20]

Empowerment is fundamentally about choices. One of the central reasons for working with patients in an empowering manner is to bring about positive change for the patient where change is the result of informed choice. However, one of the key issues that arises here centres on what is meant by 'positive change' and by 'informed'. Bringing patients to a position where they can begin to engage in making and being responsible for change in their lives and their death is not problematic for many healthcare professionals. However, there is a difference between bringing patients to a realisation that 'there is something *I* can do about my situation' and recognising that what they do is their own prerogative. The fundamental task in this regard is to ensure that patients are provided with all the relevant information and guided and supported to make what are ultimately choices and changes that they have to make and for which they *have to take responsibility*.

The very idea of empowerment is in itself problematic, as it contains the potential for either liberation from or reinforcement of exclusion. This stems from the question of whether power is something that can be bestowed as a gift/imposed as a solution, or whether it is something that can only truly be exercised by the individual or group concerned. If the first option is considered, the dilemma is easily resolved – that is, empowerment is whatever you want it to be, as it is being imposed and therefore not necessarily open to debate. However, if the approach is taken that power is best exercised by the individual or group, then a difficult, more complex and potentially more rewarding concept is developed. At this point the healthcare professional could develop the concept of full 'health' citizenship with those who are excluded, rather than simply imposing one in response to the growing tide of consumer awareness. Empowerment, then, is not the exercise of powerful conceding power as a means of managing the powerless. Empowerment is a contradiction in terms – there can only be self-empowerment. Empowerment accepts the excluded patient as a competent contributor to the design and development of strategies rather than a helpless victim with no useful assets with which to help him- or herself.

The empowerment of patients at an individual level is mainly concerned with bringing about personal change and development. It is also about providing people with the resources (information, confidence, skill, etc.) necessary to tackle the consequences of exclusion at a personal level. Within the context of palliative care it involves bringing about the control and choice of the patient's end-of-life experience. There is also a collective dimension to empowerment. This stems from the recognition that the causes of social exclusion are not to be found at the level of individuals. Therefore this empowers people to tackle the political, social and economic causes of exclusion.

As a group, therefore, patients within palliative care do hold rights. Advocacy and empowerment are a platform for a more democratic healthcare system. Self-help groups and organisations can give important signals about gaps and necessary improvements in the system. They make important contributions to a better healthcare system, which is why they should be integrated more strongly into the system.[21]

Empowering the patient who is receiving palliative care poses a difficult challenge to healthcare practitioners. Reconciling an obligation to protect whatever degree of autonomy the patient enjoys with a responsibility to promote his or her welfare will never be easy. Care must be taken not to equate age or advancement of disease with incompetence. Neither condition necessarily robs a person of all autonomy. Respect for that person requires the palliative care practitioner to persist in negotiation with him or her so that together they can make decisions which maximise the patient's welfare in every sense. A clean room in a hospice with attentive, sensitive care is not necessarily better for the patient at the end of life than a crumbling flat filled with his own possessions and the company of an equally elderly, even dirty dog – if this will enhance the individual and idiosyncratic experience of quality of life.

# Legal and non-legal responsibilities

Patient rights are a reflection of human rights. The human rights movement has gathered importance in the world since 1945 when, in the Charter of the United Nations, member states reaffirmed their faith in fundamental human rights. This was followed on 10 December 1948 by the adoption of the Universal Declaration of Human Rights, and on 4 November 1950 by the signing of the European Convention on Human Rights. After World War Two rulings of the German Supreme Court were the first in Europe to raise institutional awareness of patients' rights as citizens to be responsible for their own bodies and health, prohibiting medical treatment without consent. The rights of patients as specific human rights have only become recognised throughout the European region in the past three decades.

An important aspect of the European challenge is how to develop healthcare systems based on the values enshrined in the European Convention on Human Rights and the European Social Charter.[22] Current ongoing reforms in healthcare are mainly motivated by escalating health costs and increasing demands of the population. The question is how reforms of healthcare systems should ensure equitable access to healthcare which is both adequate and of optimal quality.

The first country in the world to introduce special patients' rights law was Finland, where a law on the patient's status and rights was passed in 1992. This law was preceded by 20 years of discussions in the Finnish Parliament. The law is administrative – that is, it contains directives which defend the provider's duties, rather than rights which the patient can demand. The second country to present patients' rights law was the Netherlands. This was part of a more extensive law reform, namely the Medical Contract Law, presented in 1995. The Dutch legislation is rights legislation for patients. Since Finland and the Netherlands have shown the way, a few other countries have introduced similar legislation, including Israel (in 1996), Lithuania (in 1996), Iceland (in 1997) and Denmark (in 1998). The Danish legislation focuses strongly on the individual and their ability to make autonomous and competent decisions in relation to their health.[23]

Until the 1970s, the health professional–patient relationship was primarily defined by the rules of medical ethics. In the following three decades the focus shifted to legal provisions, and the issue is now receiving greater international attention. The international regulations in the field of patient's rights during this time have been defined by the following legislation:

- the Universal Declaration of Human Rights (1948)
- the European Convention for the Protection of Human Rights and Fundamental Freedoms (1950)
- the European Social Charter (1961)
- the International Covenant on Civil and Political Rights (1966)
- the International Covenant on Economic, Social and Cultural Rights (1966).

In the last decade, patients' rights and citizens' empowerment have been emphasised throughout Europe. A comprehensive study of the rights of the patient in Europe was conducted in the early 1990s and was the starting point of various approaches to promote patients' rights.[24] The first international event with such a focus was the European Consultation on the Rights of Patients, convened under the auspices of the World Health Organization Regional Office for Europe (WHO/EURO) and hosted by the Government of the Netherlands in March 1994. The purpose was to define principles and strategies for promoting the rights of patients, within the context of the healthcare reform process under way in most countries. The Amsterdam consultation came at the end of a long preparatory process, during which WHO/EURO encouraged the emerging movements in favour of patients' rights by, among other things, conducting studies and surveys on the development of patients' rights throughout Europe. These studies showed a common interest and a number of policy trends and normative initiatives in the European countries, indicating that the provision of additional support for policy development in many of those countries would be appropriate. The study results were published in the book *The Rights of Patients in Europe*.[24] With the support of the Government of the Netherlands, and in broad consultation with governments and other institutions in other European countries, technical experts in the field drafted *The Principles of Patients' Rights*,[25] a comprehensive text which could be meaningful and helpful in the development of country policies on patients' rights, and which embraced the following principles:

- respect for human rights and values in healthcare
- information about health services and how best to use them
- consent
- confidentiality and privacy
- care and treatment.

The Declaration on the Promotion of Patients' Rights in Europe constitutes a common European framework for action, and includes those principles, as endorsed by the Amsterdam consultation. This declaration should be interpreted as an enhanced entitlement for citizens and patients in improving partnership in the process of care with healthcare providers and health service managers. Although no formal adoption of the declaration was envisaged, it was expected that it would be widely supported. It is perhaps significant that nearly 11 years later, it remains a document largely unknown by many palliative care practitioners. Nine years after the endorsement of the WHO/EURO Declaration on the Promotion of Patients' Rights (in Amsterdam in 1994), eight countries have enacted specific rights legislation in the spirit of the Amsterdam Declaration. These are Finland, the Netherlands, Iceland, Lithuania, Denmark, Norway, Israel and Greece.[26] A further three countries, namely France, the UK and Ireland, use a non-legal framework, the Patient's Charter, to promote the position of patients and citizens.

Next to the World Health Organization, the Council of Europe has also persistently pursued the idea of protection of the rights of patients. The Council of Europe and several non-governmental organisations (NGOs), such as the European Association of Palliative Care, Consumers International, the World Medical Association and the European Platform for Patient Organisations, Science and Industry have been involved in various activities that aim to support the development of patients' rights in Europe. The fifth conference of European Health Ministers, held in Warsaw in November 1996, had the title *Social Challenge to Health: Equity and Patients' Rights in the Context of Health Reforms*. The main purpose of the conference was to enable discussion at the highest political level of the main political, social and technical changes which are raising major concerns. These are as follows:

- the economic constraints in the face of increasing demands, particularly as a result of demographic change
- social exclusion resulting from health status
- low levels of user participation.[26]

The Ministers felt that the solution lay in a tripartite social deal between patients, providers and payers, with the commitment of all sectors and the participation of all the protagonists in order to achieve an equitable distribution. The final text adopted at the end of the debate highlighted the need for action on a number of important issues, particularly the following:

- equitable access to healthcare services by balancing the right to healthcare and financial constraints, and addressing the needs of the most disadvantaged sectors of the population
- a reassessment of the importance of health status for the social well-being of the population.

The Ministers agreed that these issues required action at the level of the individual, at the level of healthcare delivery and at government level. The attention of the Committee of Ministers was drawn to the proposal that the Council of Europe should consider building up a network for the exchange of information between member states on the following issues:

- patients' rights and patient participation
- the role of lay people in promoting health in their own environment
- the exclusion of certain groups of patients from society, in particular the chronically ill and individuals with disabilities
- the involvement of the scientific community in a setting providing treatment and procedures.

Following the Fifth Conference of Health Ministers in 1997, WHO/EURO initiated a Patients' Rights Network. The objective of this network was to support member states of the WHO European Region in their efforts to develop patients' rights legislation in accordance with the Amsterdam Declaration. Specific attention was devoted to issues such as the generic definition of the concept, negative and positive rights, legal rights, quasi rights (specifically provisions on the obligations of healthcare personnel), non-legal policy documents such as *The Patient's Charter*, and policy documents in which the right is primarily moral in nature. The name was changed to the European Partnership for Patients' Rights and Citizen Empowerment (EPPRCE).[27]

On a European level, the most recent document of greatest importance with regard to patients' rights is the *Recommendation on the Development of Structures for Citizen and Patient Participation in the Decision-Making Process Affecting Health Care*, adopted by the Council of Ministers in February 2000.[28] This Recommendation was developed in compliance with the following international documents:

- Article 11 of the European Social Charter on the Right to the Protection of Health
- Article 3 of the Convention on Human Rights and Biomedicine, requiring the Contracting Parties to provide 'equitable access to healthcare of appropriate quality', and Article 10, on the right of everyone to know any information about their health
- the Convention for the Protection of Individuals with regard to automatic processing of personal data (ETS No. 108) and Recommendation No. R (97) 5, as well as Recommendation No. R (97) 17 on the development and implementation of quality improvement systems in healthcare
- the Parliamentary Assembly of the Council of Europe on instruments of citizen participation in representative democracy (Doc. 7781(1977))
- the World Health Organization's *Health 21* programme for the European region, and its recent policy documents on patients' rights and citizens' participation
- the Amsterdam Declaration on the Promotion of Patients' Rights in Europe
- the Ljubljana Charter on Reforming Health Care, endorsed by the World Health Organization, which stresses the need for healthcare systems that focus on people and allow the 'citizens' voice and choice to influence the way in which health services are designed and operate'
- the Ottawa Charter for Health Promotion (1986) and the Jakarta Declaration on Leading Health Promotion into the Twenty-First Century (1997) as statements on the guiding principles for public health.

This was a recognition of the fact that a healthcare system should be patient-oriented and ensure the participation of citizens in decisions about their healthcare. The governments of the member states were recommended to ensure that citizens' participation applied to all aspects of the healthcare system at national, regional and local levels, and to create legal structures and policies that support citizen participation and patients' rights.

Specific guidelines were drafted which covered the following four areas.

1 *Citizen and patient participation as a democratic process*. Ensure that citizens' participation applies to all aspects of healthcare systems at national, regional and local levels. This should be observed by all healthcare system operators, including professionals, insurers and the authorities.

2 *Information*. Take steps to reflect in the law the guidelines contained in the appendix to this recommendation, and create legal structures and policies that support the promotion of citizens' participation and patients' rights, if these do not already exist.

3 *Supportive policies for active participation*. Adopt policies that create a supportive environment for the growth (in membership, orientation and tasks) of civic organisations of healthcare 'users', if these do not already exist.

4 *Participation mechanisms*. Support the widest possible dissemination of the recommendation and its explanatory memorandum, paying special attention to all individuals and organisations aiming at involvement in decision making in healthcare.

Regardless of these various initiatives and others to promote patients' rights and citizens' empowerment throughout Europe, there is a need to recognise the short-comings of using legal means to promote patient-focused legislation for palliative care. There is no golden rule on how to be successful in implementing patients' rights in a particular country. In some countries, where laws on the rights of patients have been introduced during the last decade, experience shows that legis-lation does not necessarily change the behaviour of health service personnel. One of the major problems with patients' rights legislation is the issue of implementa-tion.

This was the theme of the Thirteenth World Congress on Medical Law in Helsinki in August 2000.[29] The problem of implementation is a balance between on the one hand providing sufficient legal protection for citizens and patients, and on the other, finding acceptance and willingness with the health service personnel to respect these rights. If the healthcare professions notoriously disre-spect patients' rights, this is a signal for a present and emerging conflict between ambitions, resources and eventually values. There is a need for improved mutual understanding between legislators and health services personnel.

However, the implementation of patients' rights is not a responsibility exclu-sively for legislators and healthcare professionals. Rather, it is an obligation for all stakeholders who are involved in health services. For patient organisations, it is important that they take part in the ongoing discussion on patients' rights and invite members as well as non-members to take part in a dialogue not only to provide information on recent developments, but also to learn from their experience. At a professional level, the importance of education should not be underestimated.

Public health law is more or less unknown in Europe, except in the field of contagious diseases. However, this concept is known and generally accepted in the USA, where it is often connected to research at Schools of Public Health. Researchers in public health law are engaged in ethical conflicts of law, medicine and human rights at large. Because of the growing influence of law in healthcare services across Europe, it is important for law schools and Schools of Public Health to find ways to collaborate and to include public health law in basic training as well as in the continuous education curricula of health services personnel. To facilitate the recent need for changes in health legislation and patients' rights, it is necessary to modify the training curricula so as to provide health professionals with a solid knowledge of patients' rights legislation and policy statements. This would also serve as an important indicator of the significance of the issue. Even if several countries have introduced patients' rights laws, or are in the process of doing so, health legislation and patients' rights are not yet included to an adequate extent in the basic education and training of health professionals. At a European level, efforts can be made to further enhance the legal position of the patient. Increasing the status of the World Health Organization Declaration would support efforts to promote patients' rights and send a clear message to anyone involved in healthcare to respect the autonomy of patients.

- **A first step** would be to improve the coordination of actions taken by the World Health Organization, the Council of Europe and the European Union. This would enable these organisations to make better use of their funding and political lobbying power.
- **A second step** would be to support and organise patient organisations at a European level to meet and exchange experiences from their respective fields of expertise. The European Platform for Patients and Organisations, Science and Industry is a good example of such a forum, which will hopefully stimulate arrangements for sub-regional meetings in various regions of Europe.
- **A third step** would be to arrange a conference at ministerial level. This would focus the attention of health decision makers throughout Europe not only on the significance of new patients' rights, but also on the implementation of already existing legislation. Even if the present Declaration only deals with the *promotion* of patients' rights, this document is often referred to as one of the most important in terms of elaborating legislation and policy.

When a palliative care practitioner is engaged in caring for a patient at the end of their life, it may not seem self-evident that professional and moral responsibilities should be directed at national or international forums. There is an intimacy and sensitivity within the therapeutic and moral enterprise of palliative care that at first glance seems to be at odds with the style and purpose of ministerial debate. The palliative care practitioner *must* deliver his or her skills and care within the context of that society. This means advocating for the individual as well as the generic patient. Advocacy is the moral obligation and duty to speak out.

> *When Hitler attacked the Jews I was not a Jew, therefore I was not concerned.*
>
> *And when Hitler attacked the Catholics, I was not a Catholic, and therefore I was not concerned.*
>
> *And when Hitler attacked the unions and the industrialists, I was not a member of the unions and I was not concerned.*
>
> *Then Hitler attacked me and the Protestant church – and there was nobody left to be concerned.*[30]

The patients of palliative care practitioners are frequently those who are least able to debate and speak out at national and international forums. Feelings of hopelessness (why bother?), and the reality of vague letters, meetings and telephone calls may be emotionally, physically and spiritually beyond them. However, they are not beyond the capabilities of the professions that deliver palliative care. The delivery of palliative care does not simply occur within the context of that relationship with one patient – it is how it is seen, respected and understood by that society.

# The process of advocacy within palliative care

> *The relevance of empowerment to the ... patient is easily understood by examining the concept of power/powerlessness. Powerlessness is a common phenomenon among ... patients.... The ... patient is often the passive recipient of information and guidance from health professionals, and soon comes to consider his/her ... options and experiences as being irrelevant. Patient empowerment requires that the patient be fully informed about ... options and feel capable of participating in the decision-making about*

*these options. Further, the patient would have the ability to resist pressure from health professionals to select a specific option, and have the interpersonal skills and understanding of the medical system necessary to ensure that the selected treatment option is the one that is performed.*[31]

There is no one typical way to respond to palliative care needs. Patients will respond differently. There can be a range of emotions, ranging at once from fear, sadness or even anger to motivation and determination, and a feeling of loss of control. One way to support the patient in regaining control is to provide information that is relevant to them in a manner that is accessible.

Roberts *et al.*[32] view powerlessness in the healthcare encounter as an absence of control. In their study of the effects on a small group of patients of negotiated and non-negotiated nurse–patient interactions, they found that patients in the negotiated group reported levels of increased control on decisions occuring within the interactions than did subjects who engaged in a non-negotiated approach. The feeling of control was a function of the interactive approach with the caregiver, and was not based on the subject's personality alone. Although the study did not show that the perception of empowerment affected agreement with treatment, it was suggested that healthcare practitioners could, by increasing the patient's responsibility for and involvement in their care, be instrumental in improving patient compliance and satisfaction. Empowerment would seek to address the complexity of psychological factors implicated in decision making which arise from, and could be remedied through, the dynamics of power. For instance, the theory of learned helplessness casts light on the inhibition of human action through historical explanation of lack of control, and of negative consequences following attempts to gain control.

Empowerment goes beyond the idea of self-determination and patient autonomy in that it recognises the need for individuals to have access to the resources, including effective support, that are needed to effect their own control. The empowerment and advocacy approach is based on a range of simple ideas and tasks.

1  Include your patient in the process.
2  Do not try to manipulate them to reach the goal. Offer alternatives.
3  Encourage your patient to continue the process of listing, brainstorming and developing new options (life change/options/palliative care).
4  Encourage your patient to choose and pursue the goals that seem most important to them right now.
5  Ask your patient how you, the healthcare practitioner, can support them in achieving their own self-chosen goals, and do exactly as they request.

Life-limiting illness and the commencement of the dying process can be physically, emotionally and spiritually disempowering. The most sensitive and empathic of palliative care practitioners may still be met by a patient who is unengaged, unmotivated, and unwilling or unable to take control. Advocacy in this context is not to 'force' autonomous decision making on to a vulnerable patient who is seeking assistance, but rather to embrace the moral process of interdependence. Facilitating empowerment and demonstrating advocacy involves establishing and implementing what is important to the patient – however small or subtle that might be. It involves encouraging the patient to realise that although they may have commenced their death, choices still remain which can inform the quality of their life, and of their dying. A patient who is close to death is still a person with needs, wants and desires. The skill and art of palliative care lie in resolving those needs.

# Conclusion

The main aim of advocacy is to empower patients and carers – to help people to be heard and ensure that what they say influences the decision-making process. Patients' interests in having greater control over the process of their palliative care are real and pressing. Non-involvement and paternalistic action on the part of the healthcare practitioner can leave individuals feeling angry and resentful, particularly if they feel that they have been denied the opportunity to take responsibility and control.

In 1989, the European Association of Palliative Care published the following definition of palliative care, which was subsequently endorsed by the World Health Organization:

> *Palliative care is the active, total care of patients at a time when their disease is no longer responsive to curative treatment and when control of pain, of other symptoms and of social, psychological and spiritual problems is paramount.*
>
> *Palliative care affirms life and regards dying as a natural process; it neither hastens nor postpones death. It offers a support system to help the patient live as actively as possible until death and help the family cope during the patient's illness and in bereavement. Palliative care is multidisciplinary in its approach and encompasses the patient, the family and the community in its scope.*[33]

This definition of palliative care argues that care cannot be given in the absence of advocacy or empowerment, as it is predicated upon these. Palliative care is undertaken *with* the patient, not *to* the patient. Empowerment is a process that leads to increased personal control over one's life, however short that life may be. Empowerment-based care needs to focus on increasing each patient's participation both politically and individually.

Since understanding is the fundamental basis of decision making, information and knowledge are the two main pillars of the patient's involvement. A well-informed patient, given time and a trusting relationship with the healthcare professional, is capable of taking sound decisions about his or her health and care.

# References

1 Onions CT (ed.) (1964) *The Shorter Oxford Dictionary of Historical Principles*. Clarendon Press, Oxford.
2 Clouser KD and Gert B (1999) A critique of principalism. In: J Lindemann Nelson and H Lindemann Nelson (eds) *Meaning and Medicine: a reader in the philosophy of health care*. Routledge, London.
3 Dworkin G (1988) *The Theory and Practice of Autonomy*. Cambridge University Press, Cambridge.
4 Hill TE Jr (1991) *Autonomy and Self-Respect*. Cambridge University Press, Cambridge.
5 Veatch R (1981) *A Theory of Medical Ethics*. Basic Books, New York.
6 Beauchamp TL and Childress JF (2001) *Principles of Biomedical Ethics* (5e). Oxford University Press, Oxford.
7 Gillon R (1986) *Philosophical Medical Ethics*. John Wiley & Sons, Chichester.
8 Somerville M (1980) *Consent to Medical Care*. Law Reform Commission of Canada, Ottawa.
9 Freenan D (1996) Capacity to decide about medical treatment. *Br J Hosp Med.* **56**: 295–7.
10 Seedhouse D (1989) *Liberating Medicine*. John Wiley & Sons, Chichester.
11 Rawls J (1985) Justice as fairness: political not metaphysical. *Phil Public Affairs.* **14**: 223–51.
12 Putnam RA (1995) Why not a feminist theory of justice? In: M Nussbaum and J Glover (eds) *Women, Culture and Development: a study of human capabilities*. Clarendon Press, Oxford.
13 Little MO (1999) Why a feminist approach to bioethics? In: J Lindemann Nelson and H Lindemann Nelson (eds) *Meaning and Medicine: a reader in the philosophy of health care*. Routledge, London.
14 Baier A (1987) The need for more than justice. In: M Hanen and K Nielson (eds) *Science, Morality and Feminist Theory*. University of Calgary Press, Calgary.

15 Gregor M (ed.) (1991) *The Metaphysics of Morals. Part 2. The doctrine of virtue.* Cambridge University Press, Cambridge.

16 Feste C (1992) A practical look at patient empowerment. *Diabetes Care.* **15**: 922–5.

17 Adams R (1990) *Self-Help, Social Work and Empowerment.* Macmillan, Basingstoke.

18 Holland J, Ramazanoglu C, Scott S, Sharpe S and Thompson R (1992) Pressure, resistance, empowerment: young women and the negotiation of safer sex. In: P Aggleton, P Davies and G Hart (eds) *AIDS: rights, risk and reason.* Falmer Press, London.

19 Maclean A (1995) Empowerment and the psychiatric consumer/ex-patient movement in the United States: contradictions, crisis and change. *Soc Sci Med.* **40**: 1053–71.

20 Ornish D (1996) *Reversing Heart Disease.* Ivy Books, New York.

21 Ward D and Mullender A (1991) Empowerment and oppression: an indissoluble pairing for contemporary social work. *Critical Social Policy.* **11**: 21–30.

22 Council of Europe (1950) *Convention for Protection of Human Rights and Fundamental Freedoms.* Council of Europe, Rome.

23 Vienonen M (1999) *Why patients' rights?* Keynote address at *Patients' Rights and Citizens' Empowerment: through visions to reality.* Joint consultation between the WHO Regional Office, the Nordic Council of Ministers and the Nordic School of Public Health, Copenhagen, 22–23 April 1999.

24 Leenen HJJ, Gevers SS and Pinet G (1993) *The Rights of Patients in Europe: a comparative study.* Kluwer Law and Taxation Publishers, Deventer.

25 *The Principles of Patients' Rights*; www.inserm.fr/ethique/Ethique.nsf/397fe8563d75f39bc12563f (accessed 12 March 2003).

26 Council of Europe (1996) *Health and Quality of Life.* Fifth Conference of European Health Ministers, Warsaw, 7–8 November 1996.

27 Stachenko S (1999) *Patients' rights networks.* Keynote address at *Patients' Rights and Citizens' Empowerment: through visions to reality.* Joint consultation between the WHO Regional Office, the Nordic Council of Ministers and the Nordic School of Public Health, Copenhagen, 22–23 April 1999.

28 Council of Europe, Council of Ministers (2000) *Recommendation No. R (2000) 5 of the Committee of Ministers to member states on the development of structures for citizen and patient participation in the decision-making process affecting health care.* Adopted by the Committee of Ministers on 24 February at the 699th meeting of the Ministers' Deputies.

29 World Association for Medical Law (2000) *Thirteenth Congress of Medical Law*, Helsinki, 6–10 August.

30 Niemöller M (1968) *Holocaust Congressional Record.* p. 31636. Washington, DC. www.holocaust-history.org (accessed 22 March 2005).

31 Iverson DC, Sahay TB and Ashbury FD (1995) Personal empowerment: strategies to develop and evaluate interventions. In: *Proceedings of the International Health Promotion Conference.* Brunel University, London.

32 Roberts SJ, Krouse HJ and Michaud P (1995) Negotiated and non-negotiated nurse–patient interactions. *Clin Nurs Res.* **4**: 67–78.

33 World Health Organization (1990) *Cancer Pain Relief and Palliative Care. Report of a WHO Expert Committee.* Technical Report Series No. 804. World Health Organization, Geneva.

# 6 How informed can consent be?

## Calliope Farsides

'Consent' is a positive buzz word within healthcare vocabulary. There is usually taken to be a strong moral case for acquiring the consent of the patient, even in those areas where the legal imperative is not decisive. However, it is important to ask why consent is valued in this way, and to enquire as to the role it is meant to play in protecting and pursuing the good of the patient. It is also important to make clear what is required for consent truly to have been given, and to assess in the light of this whether there may be cases in which it is justifiable to work with something other than a clear expression of the patient's consent.

It is a regrettable fact that from the patient's perspective consent is often understood primarily as a legal mechanism designed to protect the interests of doctors. It is possible that this understanding will become increasingly prevalent, given the growing rates of litigation within the health service. Of course, consent does serve a legal function, and part of that function is to protect carers against claims that they have acted without permission, thereby becoming liable for an action in battery, or that they have failed to disclose crucial information, thereby laying themselves open to a claim of negligence. There have been a number of landmark cases involving consent, and many believe that the decisions therein have supported the doctor's position over that of the patient. When a respected legal commentator such as Professor Margaret Brazier concludes that in terms of legal attitudes to consent 'the English courts seem to say that patients must accept and acquiesce in a degree of medical paternalism many enlightened doctors now reject', it becomes apparent that on this issue at least, the law and morality might require different standards of practice.[1]

For this reason it would be more useful for present purposes to consider consent not as a primarily legal concept, but as a moral one. Raanon Gillon has provided a very useful definition which manages to capture the essential moral features of a valid consent. According to Gillon, consent is:

*a voluntary uncoerced decision made by a sufficiently competent or autonomous person, on the basis of adequate information and deliberation, to accept rather than reject some proposed course of action which will affect him or her.*[2]

By defining consent in this way, Gillon not only draws attention to the type of individual who can be reasonably expected to participate in a consenting process (i.e. a sufficiently competent person), but he also specifies the type of decision they must reach (i.e. a voluntary and deliberate choice) and the basis upon which this should be reached (i.e. in the light of adequate information, after careful deliberation, and in the absence of any form of coercion). This definition therefore places demands on carers, institutions and patients. The carer must impart sufficient information and refrain from any words or deeds which might coerce the patient or erode their voluntariness. The institution must allow sufficient time and resources to facilitate the provision of information, and provide the opportunity for reflection and deliberation. The patient must listen to the information provided and reach a decision. However, there are many respects in which this ideal might be difficult to achieve.

Let us consider first the possibility of coercion. To use an extreme example, it would be one thing for me to ask you to agree to give me a large sum of money while we were sitting together over a friendly dinner, and quite another if I (as a stranger) were to do so with a gun pointed at your head. In the first case you would probably respond to my rather unexpected request by asking me why I needed the money, and would then decide whether to give it to me, based on an evaluation of my reasons and of our friendship. In the second case you would simply respond to my threat, fearing the consequences of not doing so.

This might at first appear to be miles away from a medical or nursing scenario, but in many ways the comparison can hold. In some care settings the request for consent will be made in a way that encourages questions, gives time for reflection and allows the patient to decline. In others, a rushed and unfriendly approach will leave the patient feeling that they have no choice but to agree. The context in the sense of the physical building and arrangements might also have an effect, just as the open restaurant is quite different to a dark alley. When a person is physically comfortable and at ease, they are far less likely to be intimidated or coerced into agreeing to something with which they are unhappy. On the other hand, if they are embarrassed, uncomfortable, intimidated or distressed by their surroundings, their autonomy may well be compromised. However, the most important contextualising issue is that of the relationship between the carer who requests consent and the patient. If a friend asks me to agree to something,

I have an understandable context within which to place the request, whereas if a stranger asks me to agree to something, I have no such terms of reference. This is an issue that merits further attention.

To attach importance to the notion of consent is to characterise the relationship between patient and carer in a particular way. Of course it would not be helpful to employ the friend analogy too forcibly, but it is important to understand that some elements of that type of relationship need to be present – most obviously trust, reciprocity and beneficence. One way to represent these ideas is by presenting the relationship between carer and patient as contractual – not in the legal sense, but rather in the moral sense which implies the mutual recognition of a set of reciprocal duties and obligations adopted in the interests of pursuing shared goals. The thinking goes something like this.

By consenting to be my patient you accept that there are certain things that I may expect to do to you, and ask of you, that others would or could not. I make these claims only because we have entered a contract designed to facilitate our shared goal of pursuing your good and promoting your interests. However, simply agreeing to be my patient does not settle the consent issue once and for all. Although it might be construed as tacit permission for certain procedures and interventions, others will require your express consent, given or withheld after a specific consideration of the matter at hand.

Sometimes this consent will have a distinctly legal complexion to it (e.g. if you require surgery), but on other occasions it will be a matter of personal negotiation and understanding between you and I (e.g. when deciding between various treatment options). Your consent is a sign of your trust in me. My request for consent is a sign of my respect for you and your autonomy.

There are a number of features of this account which require further attention. First, consider the technical distinction that is often made between express and tacit consent. To consent expressly is to clearly indicate verbally or perhaps in writing that you agree to a proposed course of action. This is the clearest sign of consent, although one has to resist the idea that a verbal or written declaration is always a true sign of consent. For example, a signature at the end of a form which has been given in the absence of any explanation is not consent as morally understood. Similarly, a verbal agreement given by someone who feels too intimidated to contradict the views of the doctor is not consent in the sense that we wish to understand it here.

Because tacit consent is less clear-cut in terms of its expression, it is more open to misinterpretation, or rather we are sometimes too ready to assume its existence. Often we work on the assumption that we are entitled to assume that consent has been given when patients appear to co-operate, or at least do not complain. However, there is a level of debate over what kind of actions indicate consent in this way, and how much we can allow to be covered by tacit rather than express consent.

When I enter a doctor's surgery, it may be assumed that I tacitly consent to answer basic questions about my health state which will facilitate a diagnosis, but it should not also be assumed that I tacitly consent to remove all my clothes without an explanation of why this is necessary, nor would it be taken as consent for an invasive procedure such as a biopsy. However, this is not to suggest that express consent is only required for invasive or unusual practices. It may be the case that current practices which appear innocuous and perhaps even trivial would benefit from being re-evaluated in the light of a discussion of consent.

Consider an analogy which hopefully highlights the dangers of assuming too much. If you went to the bank to cash a cheque and handed over your cheque card which had printed upon it your full name – Mr James Bowlby – you would be somewhat surprised if the teller handed it back to you saying 'There you go, Jimmy, be a good boy and take it over to the cashier at desk number four.' Convention dictates that when names are used in such a setting, formal titles are appropriate.

However, if you find yourself in a hospital bed, hospital staff from the consultant through to the ward orderly may feel entitled to call you by whatever diminutive pet name they choose. Some patients will be unconcerned or maybe even comforted by this level of informality, while others will find it demeaning and invasive, and interpret it as a lack of respect. The point is that the convention is at odds with ordinary practice, and it has the potential to upset or insult the patient, yet rarely if ever will the question of how you wish to be addressed be raised.

It would appear that in this case it is wrong to assume tacit consent, and that the issue of how one is addressed needs to be negotiated and the patient's preference respected. Perhaps this seems a trivial point, but consider it from the opposite perspective. Imagine the surprise of the eminent consultant Professor Patricia Callow when she is suddenly beckoned across the ward by the new patient in bed number four shouting 'Hey Trish, can you toddle over here, love?'. It is highly likely that this encounter will colour the relationship that develops from then on between carer and patient, but without knowing something of the character and preferences of the professor, we cannot predict whether those effects will be good or bad. In fact, the prevailing conventions will make such an encounter unlikely and in practice rare, whereas the patient on the other hand is subject to conventions which can lead towards what they might consider patronising and irritating familiarity.

The underlying rule is this – tacit consent should be taken to mean the same as express consent, with only the mode of expression being different. Some conventions will be so widely accepted and acceptable that tacit consent to their adoption can be assumed, and the onus would be on the patient to ask that something different happen. However, in the example cited here we should remain wary of tacit consent. If we were to transport the widely acceptable convention of addressing people formally on first meeting to the hospital ward, some people would feel happy to say 'Please call me Jim' if that is what they preferred, while others would not but would nonetheless feel uncomfortable with the formality, or perhaps take it to be representative of a gap between patient and carer that does not in reality exist. Far better surely to negotiate at the outset, 'Mr Bowlby, welcome to Ward Ten. I'm Nurse Jones, but please call me Rachel if you prefer. Tell me, how would you like to be addressed while you are here?'. This will hopefully mark the beginning of the type of relationship that is required for the proper working of the contractual model of care.

Another feature of Gillon's definition that obviously requires attention is the issue of 'sufficient information'. This is commonly understood to imply a responsibility on the part of the carer to impart information to the patient. However, before considering this more familiar aspect of the issue, it is worth looking at it in a slightly different way. A morally defensible consenting process also requires the carer to collect or receive sufficient information from the patient.

The contractual model as presented here is predicated upon the assumption of shared goals. This is not contentious at a very general level – we can assume that the patient wants to be helped by the carer and that the carer wishes to help the patient. But of course we need to verify that the goals are not only shared in this general way, but also understood in the same way when it comes to specifics. What type of help does the patient want and what type of help can and will the carer offer?

This is a particularly important issue within the context of palliative care, where the carer will possibly play a major role in what is left of the patient's life and indeed their death. A patient may have particular ideas about how they wish to live the rest of their life, how they want to die, etc., and these beliefs and attitudes will be an expression of their autonomy. By understanding consent as an ongoing procedure rather than a number of single events, one facilitates the discovery of these goals and attitudes. To know that a patient still consents to the care which they are receiving requires an ongoing dialogue about and around that care and the goals that it is designed to achieve. It also requires the carer to provide the patient with information, assess their satisfaction, and listen to what they are being told. Prior to engaging in this dialogue the carer may have a very clear idea of their professional role, what they are required to do for their patient and what they are not prepared to do. However, the carer's attitudes might also have to be modified in the light of a new understanding of the goals that this particular patient has set, and the way in which this particular person evaluates the quality and value of their life.

During the course of this dialogue there may be moments when matters become complicated if, for example, the patient requests something that the carer feels unable to provide, or the patient refuses something that the carer feels obliged to offer and inclined to promote. However, the best chance of resolving these issues surely lies in establishing a full understanding between patient and carer of the goods which each is seeking to pursue. Ideally this shared knowledge would facilitate a level of tolerance and understanding which would on occasions allow one party to consent to or refuse something which is nonetheless at odds with their basic ideas.

So, for example, when exploring a patient's reasons for refusing treatment a physician might come to understand and thereby accept that this choice is appropriate for the patient, given their assessment of their quality of life, their sense of personal identity and their preferences regarding the manner and time of their death. The carer could therefore consent to the patient's request not to be treated by various means even if they themselves remained convinced that the patient's life could be maintained with a decent quality. Similarly, the patient could come to understand why the carer wanted to continue in a particular way.

Other cases might be more difficult. Consider Case study 6.1.

---

## Case study 6.1

Dillon is a traveller who hit the road three years ago, shortly after his diagnosis of testicular cancer. His philosophy of life is highly individualistic, and his past refusal of treatment means that an essentially treatable cancer has been allowed to spread. He is now in severe pain and has finally approached a local GP who has referred him to you at the local pain control clinic based within the hospice. Dillon has requested pain control, but refuses to accept the particular drugs you are recommending because he claims they are made by a 'particularly immoral' pharmaceutical company. You believe that the company is no worse than any other – in fact in many respects they have a good record. However, you trust that Dillon will not have any knowledge of a smaller company that produces a near equivalent, and although you know them to have been involved in rather shady dealings in the developing world, you prescribe their drug and keep quiet. Dillon agrees to take the drugs.

In this example it is probably very difficult for the doctor to understand the patient and to share their value systems. However, the doctor appears to find a way to make Dillon feel all right about his actions, even if they are essentially no better than the choice he rejected. His may be the best course of events in one respect, but we need to ask whether Dillon has really consented and whether his values have been respected. It might be that no drug has yet been produced by means that Dillon considers to be ethical, and if we were truly to respect his position we would need to allow him to refuse all mainstream therapies. This would be a very difficult option for many carers to accept, but it would show respect for the autonomy of a patient who would appear to be competent to make decisions about his life and welfare, and the values that he wishes to live by.

However, in the past and still to an extent today there has been a readiness on the part of healthcare practitioners to substitute their own perceptions of what constitutes good for those of the patient, or to pursue their conception of the goals of medicine unquestioningly, assuming them to be universally endorsed. This is essentially paternalism, and one of the functions of consent is to guard against the excesses of paternalism. In imparting the information necessary to consent, one allows the patient to either share or contradict one's view, and if they wish to do so they can make it their own. In discovering important information about the patient one is forced to acknowledge that their world view might be radically different to one's own, and that this will have consequences for the choices that they make.

However, there may be justified forms of paternalism that are appropriate to the care of particular patients, and a feature of some justifiable forms of paternalism may well be the willingness to act in the patient's best interest irrespective of their consent. This is an issue in the treatment of those who are judged incompetent to give consent. However, it might also be an issue where the costs to the patient of being asked to give consent are thought to be too great.

Consider the following case.

## Case study 6.2

Jean is a 42-year-old woman with breast cancer. She is aware of her diagnosis and prognosis, but she has said from the outset that she cannot take
responsibility for her treatment in any way. She does not wish to be made
to choose between options, but rather she wants you to decide on her
behalf. She is happy to hear from you why you decided to make the
choices you have made, and to that extent she will be fully informed of
the situation. In this case consent has been given for the carer to take
complete control of the management of the patient. Jean remains perfectly
happy with the arrangement, and devotes her time to sorting out those
things that she thinks matter most in the time she has left.

Such an arrangement places a heavy responsibility on the carers, but it may be
one that they should be prepared to accept on behalf of some patients.
However, for it to work properly the carers not only need to know of all the
necessary information about the care they can offer, but they also need to know
Jean, as this will be the only way to ensure that the choices they make on her
behalf are appropriate and, looking at it from the opposite angle, that is what
they have consented to do. Some would object to this arrangement, as it pays
too little attention to patient autonomy, but this need not be the only interpretation.

Consent often indicates trust, and allows the patient to hand over control and
responsibility without losing autonomy. Autonomy is usually defined and understood in terms of the idea of self-rule, and is taken to be a particularly valuable
feature of humanity which should be promoted and respected. It is thought to be
intrinsically good to be master of one's own life, and further extrinsic good is
taken to follow on from this. However, it is important not to confuse autonomy
with a crude notion of substantive independence. There are times in one's life
when one does not wish to be entirely in control of one's welfare, and in fact
no great benefit would follow from being so. Others are the experts on the issue
in question, and to hand over some control to them would be of benefit both in
terms of securing the best outcome, and also in terms of relieving oneself of
responsibilities that one might not feel equipped to fulfil.

The crucial term here is *hand over*, and one can add to this the idea of
consenting to do so, and monitoring and reassessing one's decision over time.
If I consent to allow someone to take control of some important aspect of my

life, then my autonomy is not eroded, even though my level of independence
and control has been. If I employ an expert accountant to take care of my financial affairs, I consider this to be quite different to an overbearing partner
insisting on doing so. I employ the accountant because of their expertise, and I
understand them to be relieving me of an onerous burden. My partner, on the
other hand, in denying me control without my agreement attacks my autonomy.
If the accountant were to decide to take radical action which went beyond the
normal duties I understood her to be carrying out, then I might believe that she
also was taking too much control, and I would feel that my autonomy was
being threatened.

Consent is an ongoing process, with only a limited range of activities taken to
be tacitly consented to once the original relationship is set up. Not everyone is
like Jean, nor should they be treated in the manner that she requests. Care
should generally be seen as shared rather than delegated, negotiated rather than
prescribed.

Many of the features of Gillon's definition underline the importance of time in
the consenting process, and lack of time needs to be acknowledged as a potential
problem. Time is needed for the patient to be assessed with regard to their
competence, and time is also needed for information to be given, understood
and deliberated on. Time is needed to form the relationship between carer and
patient which will protect against the dangers of coercion and unjustified paternalism. Time is also important because, over time, circumstances relevant to
consent can change.

Consider the relationship between a GP and a patient. If you see the same GP
from childhood, at a certain point the terms of the relationship will need to be
renegotiated. When you are very young, your parents act as proxies and give
their consent to treatment as required. As you get older they do not need to
fulfil this role, and it should not be assumed that you consent to your parents
being involved with or even informed of your medical treatment. As you reach
old age, or in specific situations before then, the need for a proxy might arise
again, or at least there might be occasions on which it is wise to keep another
person informed of your situation. With this in mind, carers will need to
constantly check back to establish who are the significant others in the picture
and the extent to which they may be consulted or informed, if at all.

Likewise, in a relationship that exists over time, the doctor's understanding of
the attitudes and beliefs of the patient needs to be reconfirmed over time, and
sometimes issues need to be raised and discussed in anticipation of later events
or conditions that the patient might experience. For example, a GP should not
assume that a child will share the moral beliefs of his or her parents, or that a

person who was vehemently opposed to something in early life remains similarly committed at a later stage.

But of course few of us enjoy the luxury of continuous care as characterised by the old-style family doctor. On the cancer journey our care might pass through many hands and we might confront many different types of institution. Yet at each point along the way it is important for the carers to know who we are, where we have come from and where we wish to go. An important aspect of early outpatient care might be not only to discuss with patients the issues that are important to their later care management and treatment choices, but also to share with them their understanding of the situation in which they find themselves and the continuities and discontinuities with their earlier life.

The key to successful consent throughout the therapeutic relationship lies with the successful establishment and nurturing of the relationship between carer and patient, and the sharing of information, ideas, plans and goals that they discuss together over time. The time available will of course vary depending upon when and how a person is diagnosed and what type of care they have access to. Continuity of care over time offers the fullest opportunities for information sharing, understanding and consent, but it should be possible for a patient's care to pass successfully through the hands of different people, so long as those carers work together to ensure that the patient experiences the same essential relationship with each of them.

Consider the following case.

## Case study 6.3

Rachel has been attending the local hospice as an outpatient for two years since she was first diagnosed with non-Hodgkin's lymphoma. She has seen Ian, the nurse manager of the unit, on each of her regular visits. They have discussed many things together, not always matters related to her illness, and Ian has kept a full set of notes documenting what he considers to be significant information emerging from their conversations. At the beginning of each visit Ian shares these notes with Rachel, and she confirms whether they were an accurate account of what was said or understood. Unfortunately, Rachel is now quite ill and confined to her home, where Susie the community nurse visits her regularly. With Rachel's agreement, Susie has read through Ian's notes and has discussed them with Rachel on her second visit.

Ian's notes give Susie an initial introduction to her patient, and allow Rachel to build a relationship with Susie without having to rebuild the basic foundations. Future consents will be informed by numerous previous discussions between Ian and Rachel, even though Ian is no longer directly involved in her care. The other side of the coin is that Susie has a responsibility to make Rachel feel happy with her, and to get to know her in the relatively short time they might have together.

Having moved away from the old misconception that 'there is nothing more we can do' once a person is found to be terminally ill, there are increasing numbers of therapeutic options available designed to either prolong or improve the quality of that life. However, some of these treatments are in themselves burdensome, and it is not always clear that the right choice would be to intervene. Yet, if such treatments are available and there is at least some chance of improvement, one could say that to fail to disclose the possibility of benefit and offer the patient a choice is unduly paternalistic.

The problem is that in order to facilitate rational choice one has to give the patient all of the relevant facts, some of which will be difficult to cope with, while others can only be presented as possibilities or probabilities. Furthermore, to make choices which affect their future, the patient needs to understand what their future holds for them, and that might be knowledge that they have so far chosen to resist acquiring. The lesson here is that the possibility of choice and the need to gain consent require openness and honesty through the course of the entire relationship between carer and patient. If these have always been features of this relationship, the particular truths that have to be delivered at moments of choice will not come as a shock in the same way as they might when a carer has paternalistically selected what the patient should or should not know.

At the end of life a person might no longer be competent or able to make decisions or express their consent. This does not mean that there will not be important choices to be made, nor does it mean that consent can or should disappear from the picture. There are a number of different ways in which consent can still be incorporated in such a patient's care. First, following on from the discussion above, it should be possible for carers and patients to work together and discuss in advance the types of choices a person would want to make in given situations. This is formalised by way of the advance directive or living will.

Consider the following case.

## Case study 6.4

Robert is a 42-year-old gay man suffering from end-stage HIV-related disease. He is blind, barely conscious and mildly demented. However, he can be cared for easily at home and has as yet required no unusual means to keep him alive. His partner David has cared for him devotedly and now feels that it is time for him to die before his dignity is eroded further. Robert's mother agrees and is happy to care for him alongside David. However, Robert's father and sister feel that he should be admitted to hospital so that 'something could be done' were a crisis to occur. Robert has prepared a living will, but actually found that he could live with some of the conditions he previously considered intolerable, such as his blindness. Therefore, although still competent, he chose not to activate it.

Such a case hints at the problems associated with remaining true to the moral purpose of consent once a patient is no longer competent. An advance directive is a form of prospective consent expressly given. In such a document the patient will avail of their legal right to specify what types of treatments and interventions they wish to refuse at what stage in their life. There are a number of difficulties with these documents, and it is rare for them not to require some form of interpretation or endorsement by others. However, combined with an understanding of the patient based on earlier encounters, or through discussion with significant others, it should be possible to ascertain when, if at all, it is appropriate to activate such a document, and thereby to let the patient effectively consent while they are non-competent.

Prior to the development of these documents the only options were proxy consent, hypothetical consent (deciding on the basis of what someone would consent to if only they were able), or beneficent management in the interests of the patient. Each of these options raises problems. In the case of Robert we would need to ask who should act as proxy. Is it the person with the firmest legal relationship, or the person closest to and most cognisant of the patient's wishes? Should those who have the clearest legal right to decide necessarily enforce that right against others who would be better qualified to decide on behalf of the patient?

The problem is that all those gathered at the bedside love Robert and want to do what is best for him, and it is difficult to admit that one might not be the best person to judge what precisely that is. David feels that what is best for Robert at this stage is 'what Robert wants', but Robert is unable to tell us, so we need to work it out. David will do this by referring back to discussions they have had since Robert's diagnosis, by recalling the way he has seen Robert live his life, and the plans he knows Robert to have made for his death. The problem is that Robert has already abandoned one of the plans he earlier made, and we have no way of knowing how he feels at the moment. Robert's father and sister may see the best for Robert as 'more life', and therefore they wish to secure that on his behalf. His mother may see the best for Robert in terms of an end to his pain and suffering irrespective of what he has or has not said in the past.

Deciding what is in the patient's best interests is not the simple task it is presented as when carers suggest that, in the absence of consent, we should decide in the patient's best interest. For this reason it is in the interest of all those involved to develop the consenting process in ways that allow it to be part of a patient's care even when their competence has vanished, be that through involving the patient at an earlier stage in the appointment and briefing of proxies, or through fine-tuning the advance directive mechanism to make it a reliable expression of the patient's wishes.

This chapter has looked at the issue of consent and has indirectly tackled the question of whether it can be fully informed, but it has done so in a rather unexpected way. Of course there are important questions surrounding the issue of how much a patient should be told, when they should be told, how they should be told, and by whom. There are minimum standards which ought to be met on all these points, and there are moral and empirical arguments to support specific levels of information giving as necessary to appropriate consent. However, all of this good work will come to naught if this information is fed into a context which undermines its purpose.

Information – that is, the facts when they are available, and probabilities or opinions when they are not – is the basic raw material of deliberation and choice. Competence, autonomy and confidence provide the patient with the tools that they need in order to work with that raw material. A strong, open and truthful relationship with their carers affords them invaluable assistance in their task. Most importantly of all, the information that the carer gathers about the patient allows them to assist in the task without getting in the way, to take over the task when the patient is in difficulties and asks for help, to carry the burden when the task gets too much for the patient to bear, or to step in when the patient loses the basic skills that they need in order to progress. Consent is not always possible, nor are patients always willing to carry the responsibilities that it imposes. Plans need to be in place should these eventualities occur.

Wherever possible consent needs to be an ongoing component of care, but so does the free and honest exchange of information. Without the latter the former becomes a sham, and without either the patient at best gets lost within a sea of beneficence and at worst is drowned in professional arrogance. In order to make a rational choice the patient needs to know the relevant information, and to make a free, voluntary and uncoerced choice the patient needs to know and trust their carer. To ensure that consent is given, the carer needs to impart information to the patient and gather information about the patient in order to build the relationship that is needed to insure against coercion, intimidation or undue influence. Only when both sides of this contract are fulfilled will consent be fully informed in the way that we require it to be.

# References

1 Brazier M (1992) *Medicine, Patients and the Law*. Penguin Books, Harmondsworth.
2 Gillon R (1986) *Philosophical Medical Ethics*. John Wiley & Sons, London.

# Further reading

British Medical Association (2003) *BMJ Medical Ethics Today* (2e). BMJ Publishing Group, London.
Buchanan A and Brock D (1990) *Deciding for Others: the ethics of surrogate decision making*. Cambridge University Press, Cambridge.
Doyal L and Tobias JS (2001) *Informed Consent in Medical Research*. BMJ Books, London.
Dworkin G (1988) *The Theory and Practice of Autonomy*. Cambridge University Press, Cambridge.
Farsides B (2002) An ethical perspective – consent and patient autonomy. In: J Tingle and A Cribb (eds) *Nursing Law and Ethics*. Blackwell Science, Oxford.
McHale J (2002) Consent and the capable adult patient. In: J Tingle and A Cribb (eds) *Nursing Law and Ethics*. Blackwell Science, Oxford.
O'Neill O (2002) *Autonomy and Trust in Bioethics*. Cambridge University Press, Cambridge.

# 7 Euthanasia: slippery slope or mercy killing?

## Marney Prouse

## Introduction

It has long been thought that the process of dying is a straightforward one. Generations before ours were saddened but resigned to death as an inevitable part of life. Wilkes[1] suggests that, until recently, death was a social act. Significant technological changes now intervene to keep patients alive. The patient of the past would have followed a natural progression from illness or injury through to organ failure and death. However, the patient of today may find that technology interferes with this natural order.

David Lamb[2] writes that whereas death is an event, dying is a process. Technology fulfils Lamb's prophecy by steering the course of death so that it continues to be a process rather than a final event, and by making it a far cry from the social act that it once was. Allowing the process to play such a dominant role creates moral dilemmas for those who would have died in the past and who would now choose to die, but who find that they would need assistance in doing so.

Few subjects provoke such heated debate as euthanasia. The battle-lines are inevitably drawn between those who believe in the sanctity of life at all costs and those who believe that all individuals who are terminally ill should be free to determine the moment and route of their death. The purpose of this chapter is not to determine whether euthanasia is right or wrong, but to arm the reader with some essential ethical arguments that are both critical and challenging. Another aim is to examine some of the most debated arguments and to present some often unacknowledged alternatives to them, based on overviews of writings by a number of contributors to the field. This subject has challenged some of the greatest minds through the ages, and many books and treatises have been written as a result. This chapter will present a brief overview of some of that thinking, and hopefully will encourage the reader to explore the concepts on a fuller and deeper basis.

The logical starting point for this discussion is to define the concept. This being a complex subject, its definition is necessarily complex and not universally agreed. Glover[3] baldly states that the term 'euthanasia' is used to mean:

> *killing someone, where, on account of his distressing physical or mental state, this is thought to be in his own best interests. It is to include someone who is about to enter such a state as well as someone who is already there.*

Roy and Rapin,[4] writing on behalf of the European Association for Palliative Care, state that the term should be reserved for:

> *compassion-motivated, deliberate, rapid and painless termination of the life of someone afflicted with an incurable and progressive disease. If a suffering and terminally ill person is not allowed to die – his or her life is terminated.*

It is often on the basis of such emotive words as 'killing' and 'termination' that discussions on the subject stray into imbalance.

Some further definitions have been advanced in a report published by the House of Lords Select Committee on Medical Ethics,[5] when the sub-committee considered evidence on the subject of euthanasia. They subdivided euthanasia into three further categories.

**Voluntary euthanasia** occurs when the patient is capable of giving consent and requests his or her own death.

**Non-voluntary euthanasia** occurs when the patient does not have the capacity to understand what euthanasia means, and therefore cannot form a request or withhold consent because they have significant learning disabilities or mental illness, or are unconscious. Two major challenges emerge when dealing with patients who fall into these categories. The first is when third parties seek permission for them to die, most often through a withdrawal of treatment. The second and perhaps more critical issue is that these patients cannot give consent because they are deemed to be incompetent.

One of the first patients whose circumstances created a medico-legal dilemma, in 1976, was Karen Ann Quinlan, an American woman in persistent vegetative state (PVS) (as quoted by Pabst Battin[6]). The first person to test the judicial climate in the UK was Tony Bland, who was also in PVS for a prolonged period as a result of being injured at the Hillsborough football stadium disaster in 1993.

The issues involved in this type of euthanasia will be discussed later in the chapter.

**Involuntary euthanasia** is the killing of a patient who is capable of understanding and consenting to the act, but does not do so. This is known as murder within the ambit of the law.

**Assisted suicide** describes the act sought by a competent patient who wishes to end his or her life, but who requires assistance in order to perform the act, either because of a physical disability or, as in most cases, because the patient is not armed with sufficient information to ensure that death will be guaranteed. Physician-assisted suicide as described by the American Medical Association (AMA)[7] occurs:

> *when the physician facilitates a patient's death by providing the necessary means and/or information to enable the patient to perform the life-ending act (e.g. the physician supplies sleeping pills and information about the lethal dose while aware that the patient may commit suicide).*

**Passive euthanasia** was a term widely used to describe the withholding or withdrawing of life-sustaining treatment, by which the patient is allowed to die. The use of the term has fallen foul of the palliative care community, who have suggested that the terms 'active' and 'passive' are ambiguous and misleading and should therefore be avoided. The House of Lords Select Committee[5] agrees with the European Association of Palliative Medicine and suggests that more appropriate descriptors are 'withdrawing or not initiating treatment or ... a treatment-limiting decision'. The Dutch use the term *levesbeeindigend handelen* (life-terminating acts), that encompasses the withholding and withdrawing of all treatment. It is used to refer to the direct termination of life as found in the Remmelink Commission Report commissioned by the Dutch Supreme Court in 1991–92.[6]

# The legal status of euthanasia

The legal status of euthanasia and assisted suicide has been hotly debated by legislators and the judiciary in a number of countries, focusing on either the legalisation or the decriminalisation of the acts. The Northern Territory in Australia was the first state to legalise and sanction the practice of euthanasia, in 1996. The first case of euthanasia under that law occurred in September 1996, when a man who was terminally ill was able to commit suicide with the help of a computer-assisted lethal injection that was prepared by his general practitioner. On 24 March 1997, a bill was passed in the Australian Parliament that overturned the legality of the decision, and it currently remains illegal to practise euthanasia.[7]

In Oregon in the USA, the practice of euthanasia was legalised with the Death with Dignity Act in 1997 after a referendum was held to support its use. An immediate challenge to that law occurred, and although the law was a valid one, an appeal by opposition groups made the practice illegal immediately. The United States Supreme Court rejected the challenge to the law in 1997. Doctors were able to prescribe terminally ill patients life-ending oral drugs, but were not allowed to administer them. Statistics are not known to be reliable, although a statistical report published in March 2003[8] outlining the number of deaths under the Act reported a total of 129 over the five-year period for which the Act was in force. It is worth noting that a cause for concern is the fact that doctors are limited to prescribing oral medication under Measure 16, which may delay death, due to either regurgitation or poor absorption. On 6 November 2001, Attorney General John Ashcroft issued a directive (formerly known as the *Ashcroft Directive*) stating that a doctor could lose his or her registration if it was discovered that federal funds were used to prescribe controlled substances for the purpose of assisting a patient to commit suicide. The *Ashcroft Directive* has been the subject of lengthy and numerous court proceedings, without resolution to date, and will be heard in the US Supreme Court in its session beginning October 2005.[9]

The Netherlands legalised euthanasia in 2002, subject to safeguards and restrictions. Prior to its legalisation, euthanasia was legally tolerated and, contrary to public perception, it was considered a criminal act for a doctor or other healthcare professional to commit euthanasia in Holland. However, a healthcare professional could be protected from prosecution through a defence of necessity, assuming that there was scrupulous adherence to stringent criteria. Failure to meet the criteria could result in a maximum prison sentence of 12 years. The criteria continue to apply, and in December 2002 the Dutch Supreme Court upheld the rules relating to euthanasia by convicting a GP of assisted suicide when he assisted an elderly man who was tired of living (*see* www.inter nationaltaskforce.org/ashover.htm).

The law is clear that:

- the patient must face a future of unbearable, interminable suffering
- the consent for euthanasia must come from a competent patient alone
- the request to die must be voluntary and well considered
- the doctor and the patient must be convinced that there is no other solution

- a second medical opinion must both be obtained and life must be ended in a medically appropriate way
- the patient facing incapacitation may leave a written agreement to their death.[10]

The Netherlands Government is aware that under-reporting may be an issue, and is attempting to document to what extent euthanasia is under-reported. A written report is required for all cases of euthanasia and physician-assisted suicide. A report published in 1990 suggested that 82% of cases in that year were not reported, and in 1995 a follow-up report suggested that 59% of cases were not reported. There have been other concerns about the use of euthanasia practices for patients with depressive illnesses. Should this be a reason to invoke euthanasia or physician-assisted suicide?[11]

Assisted suicide is not a criminal act in Switzerland if it is motivated by altruistic considerations.[12] Criminal Code par. 155 (1937) Switzerland has had no law prohibiting assisted suicide since 1937, when its criminal code was revised. Since assisted suicide is legal, anyone may assist the suicide of a physically ill person for the purpose of relieving suffering. No official statistics are available. There are no safeguards and no residency requirements, and there is no investigation unless someone notifies the police.[12] A controversy was ignited in the early part of 2003 when Reginald Crew, a British man with motor neurone disease, flew to Switzerland in order to be allowed to participate in an assisted suicide under the auspices of an assisted suicide group known as Dignitas. He died as a result, and since his death there have been suggestions that his wife, who accompanied him, should be prosecuted under the Suicide Act for aiding and abetting his suicide. At the time of going to press, no further action was taken. However, the case has raised an interesting proposition about the reach of the law (remembering, of course, that Switzerland is not part of the European Union) and the challenges of so-called 'suicide tourism'.

The Belgian physician-assisted suicide law came into effect in September 2002. A permanent committee to monitor such deaths was set up. The committee must approve an official form for physicians to fill out every time they assist a suicide. A 39-year-old multiple sclerosis patient died from a lethal injection one week after the new law came into effect. Under the law a patient must request euthanasia at least one month before the killing is carried out, and a second opinion must be sought if the patient is not in the final stages of a terminal illness. Belgium's professional medical organisation has complained that the killing was illegal, and is considering whether to take legal action over the case.[12]

The legal position in the UK is clear – euthanasia is a criminal offence, although the courts have reacted by not convicting doctors under the Suicide Act since its introduction in 1961. One of the more recent cases involved a British GP being acquitted of murder when he gave lethal doses of drugs to a terminally ill cancer patient, using the doctrine of double effect (discussed below) as his defence.[10] The judge in this case stressed that the intention to relieve suffering was the primary feature of this decision, and if that was the case, then it would be lawful to administer whatever dose of drug was required to relieve the pain.

Section 2(1) of the Act states that it is an offence 'to aid, abet, counsel or procure the suicide of another or an attempt by another to commit suicide'. However, this does not stop charges being laid under the criminal law, the most common being a charge of murder. Under the same Act, it is not a crime for an individual to commit suicide by their own hand – that is, a person who is capable of committing suicide will not be considered to have committed a crime if they physically take a substance that will lead to their death. The issues become more complicated when a person must rely on someone else to assist them in taking tablets, injecting medication, etc., and this is when the criminal element emerges.

Attempts have been made to support and oppose euthanasia through the legislature. In 1997, the Doctor-Assisted Dying Bill was rejected. In 2000, the Medical Treatment (Prevention of Euthanasia) Bill 12 met with a similar fate.

The dividing line between withdrawal of treatment from an incompetent patient and involuntary euthanasia was highlighted in the House of Lords, the highest domestic court in the UK. The case of Tony Bland held that the issue of distinction was that continuation of treatment was not in his best interests. The House of Lords distinguished withdrawal of treatment from euthanasia on the grounds that withdrawing or withholding life-prolonging treatment was an omission and not a positive act to end a life. A doctor's omission could only be considered culpable under UK law if he or she was under a duty to act. The House of Lords determined that there was no duty to continue treatment.[13]

Two interesting and seemingly linked cases appeared before UK courts in the early part of the new millennium, where the 'right to die' was identified as being the key feature of both cases and has disguised vastly different legal issues. Two British women, Dianne Pretty and Ms B, both of whom had terminal illnesses, challenged the legal, societal and medical views of this complex issue by making demands upon the court to choose the time and method of their own deaths. Both women exercised what they believed to be their rights in determining their destinies, and have reawakened public awareness of a highly emotive and complicated legal decision-making process with two very different outcomes.

Ms B, a 43-year-old single former social worker, suffered an acute haemorrhage of the blood vessels in her spine, resulting in total paralysis from the neck down. She was given artificial ventilation to allow her to breathe, upon which she was completely dependent and without which she would die. For over a year she was completely dependent on full-time hospital caregivers to meet the most basic of physical needs, and she had no immediate family to care for her. Ms B prepared two separate living wills, the contents of which she brought to the attention of her treating doctors, in which she clearly expressed her wishes about not wanting to be artificially ventilated. Medical staff stated that they thought that the terms of the document were not specific enough to warrant withdrawal of treatment.

Dianne Pretty was also 43 years old, a former cook, married and a mother of two. She was severely disabled with motor neuron disease, which had resulted in complete immobility. Like Ms B, she was completely dependent on caregivers, particularly her husband, to meet her most basic needs. Until very shortly before her death she lived at home, and she moved to a hospice during the very last stage of her life.

Both women reached a point where they chose not to continue to live with their illnesses and, as a result, made applications to the courts to support their decisions to end their lives at a time and in a manner that was acceptable to them.

Ms B's application to the court was made to seek a declaration from the court that the continued unauthorised invasive treatment in the form of mechanical ventilation was a form of unlawful trespass. In effect, she was making a request to her treating doctors to turn her ventilator off, so that she would die quickly – she was refusing invasive treatment that was prolonging her life. The main issue facing the court was whether or not Ms B was mentally competent to make decisions about her treatment, even if her refusal of treatment resulted in her death. The hospital in which she was being treated was concerned that it would face prosecution if it complied with her wishes. Her doctors offered her a slow and painful alternative to switching off the ventilator that would mean it would take significantly longer for her to die, and which she resolutely refused.

Like Ms B, Dianne Pretty had also been assessed to be a mentally competent individual. Her original submission to the court was to ask the Director of Public Prosecutions to allow her husband to assist her in ending her life, as she was physically unable to perform the act herself. This request was refused, and Mrs Pretty made an application to the courts to have that decision judicially reviewed. A judicial review was held, and as a result the case was referred to the House of Lords. If Mrs Pretty had the physical capability, she would have been legally entitled to commit suicide under the Suicide Act 1961. She asked that her husband would be protected from prosecution as a person aiding and abetting a suicide under section 2(1) of the Act if he assisted her. She further argued that not allowing her to decide the time and method of her death was a violation of her rights under the European Convention on Human Rights, principally under Article 2 (the right to die as a corollary of the right to life), Article 3 (prohibition of inhuman and degrading treatment) and Article 8 (the right to respect for private and family life).

This was the first time that the House of Lords had been asked to consider a case of assisted suicide by a terminally ill individual. Dianne Pretty's application to the House of Lords was met with sympathy, but her appeal was dismissed as she was unable to effectively establish the main issue before the House of Lords, namely that the UK is in breach of the Convention by failing to permit (assisted suicide) or that it would be in breach of the Convention if it did not permit it. Mrs Pretty made an appeal to the European Court of Human Rights on the same grounds and her application was given priority, given the serious nature of her condition.

Both courts were unable to deny the value of the ethical principles of autonomy and self-determination that were central to the arguments in both cases. Beauchamp and McCullough[14] have said that:

> *The principle of self-determination means that one has sovereignty over one's life – a sovereignty that protects privacy as well as rights to control what happens to one's person and one's property.... Rights of individual sovereignty protect an individual's freedom to choose his or her best inter-ests.... Legal rights are a way of limiting the physician's power and of protecting the patient from unwarranted intrusions.*

These principles underpin the European Convention on Human Rights and, domestically, in the Human Rights Act 1998. However, public interest arguments, such as those that surround all aspects of euthanasia, seem to meet with particular resistance in the application of these rights.

It is clear that, in the case of Ms B, the principles of autonomy and self-determination have been fully supported as a right to refuse treatment as she is able to die in the manner that she chooses. But is this merely a case of semantics? The mischievous observer might ask what would happen if, instead of saying 'I do not wish to have this treatment', Ms B said 'What I really want to do is to end my life', and one of the ways to do that was to switch off her ventilator, without which she knows she would die very quickly. It is a fact that she lacks the physical capacity to perform that action, so in fact she relies on others to perform that act for her. How far removed is this from the case of Dianne Pretty, who is asking someone else to assist her?

What then is the sticking point between these seemingly similar cases? Is it because the hospital owes a duty of care to Ms B and she could demand her right to terminate treatment, whereas it could be argued that Dianne Pretty's husband as a non-medical person does not? Is it because Dianne Pretty is asking her husband to take positive steps to end her life and that Ms B is asking medical professionals to withdraw care, knowing that her rights are fully enshrined in UK law? Policy decisions undeniably acted as barriers to Dianne Pretty's case, particularly with regard to the issues of safeguards around the conduct of assisted suicide.

What do these decisions mean for the health service and for clinical care of competent patients? In the case of Ms B, the role of doctors as the ultimate decision makers and benevolent paternalists has been clearly challenged. The court was critical of the way in which this matter was handled, and felt that the clinical decision to offer an inappropriate clinical alternative 'appears to have been designed to help the treating clinicians ... and not in any way designed to help Ms B.' The court made it extremely clear that this case defined what should have been a standard part of clinical practice, and several shortcomings were highlighted. The court criticised the hospital administration for leaving this matter for too long in the hands of clinicians who were acting out of their depth. It also became clear that there were no apparent external supports available to the clinical team in the form of an ethics committee or health authority support. Despite taking legal advice on the matter, the trust failed to act decisively to reach a conclusion on the matter. As a final criticism, the court awarded Ms B nominal damages for unlawful trespass. It was noted that the trust had spent in excess of £100 000 on legal fees to dispute a matter that was exceedingly clear in law.

# The law in respect of refusal of treatment

In order to resolve any future confusion, the court set out clear practice guidelines following the case of Ms B, which are briefly summarised here. The court felt that the fundamental cornerstone of refusal of treatment lies in determining that the patient has sufficient mental capacity to make a decision of this gravity. Once this has been clearly established, adequate information and options must be available to the patient to enable him or her to make an informed decision about the future. The court went so far as to direct clinicians not to confuse mental capacity with the nature of a decision made by a patient, regardless of the consequences, even if refusal results in death. In other words, the patient's view may represent a difference in values, rather than an absence of capacity. If issues of mental capacity still exist, the team is directed to include the patient as a partner in his or her care. Finally, the hospital is charged with responsibility for resolving the issue as a matter of priority. If the matter cannot be resolved locally, then a duty exists to find a doctor who will carry out these wishes.

This raises an interesting point. Should euthanasia or assisted suicide be solely in the domain of the medical professional? Or is there a case, as in Switzerland, for allowing non-medical people to participate in the act? In order to answer this question, you must be fully armed with appropriate arguments, so there is a need to read on before answering.

Both courts highlighted the value of palliative care in the treatment of people with life-threatening illnesses, and emphasised how all avenues of care should be explored and considered before making a final decision to end life. This may be seen to be a somewhat beneficent view, but perhaps it could be defended on the grounds that consideration of this type of care fulfils the requirements for making an informed decision.

Was the weakest point in Diane Pretty's case the fact that she was not being cared for in a medical environment, and therefore not in a position of refusing treatment? The irony of both of these cases is that Ms B, although profoundly disabled, did not necessarily have a dramatically shortened life expectancy. She was able to choose the course of her life and death because she was being treated in a hospital. Dianne Pretty, on the other hand, knew that her life would end in months, if not weeks, and that she faced the prospect of a distressing death. As she was being cared for at home until the last few days of her life, she did not have the ability to refuse treatment in a way that would shorten her life. On 29 November 2001, the House of Lords unanimously rejected Diane Pretty's request for assisted suicide. The court held that the European Convention on Human Rights is in place to protect life rather than to take it. On 29 April 2002, the European Court of Human Rights upheld England's ban on assisted suicide. Diane Pretty died in May 2002. Just before she died she stated that 'the law has taken all of my rights away'.[10] Is there a moral difference between the positive commission of an act (giving tablets to end life) and an omission or failure to perform a positive act? This is your first test for developing sound arguments in the subject area.

A paper reported from Scotland in the *Lancet*[15] suggests that a distinction can be made between euthanasia and the withdrawal of treatment, and the various routes to death that are collectively, and possibly inaccurately, called euthanasia. In order to resolve this distinction, the paper suggests isolating the various aspects of the term and addressing them within the law. It should be clearly noted here that the law in Scotland is legally separated from that in England and Wales. However, the principle is a sound one. One suggestion that was made a number of years ago was to deal with persistent vegetative state as a separate entity and to propose the introduction of a Medical Futility Bill. Although this Bill did not come to fruition, the concept is an interesting one. The proposal was to develop the following wording:[16]

> It will not be unlawful to withdraw treatment, including physiological replacement therapy such as artificial ventilation and feeding, when at least two independent registered medical practitioners, one of whom must be a consultant neurologist, are of the opinion that the patient has sustained such damage to the central nervous system that:
> - he cannot exist in the absence of continuous care
> - he is permanently unable to participate in human relationships and experiences
> - continued treatment cannot improve his condition and is therefore futile
> - the patient's nearest relatives or carers have been consulted.

The authors of this proposed bill consider physician-assisted suicide and suggest that as suicide has never been a criminal offence in Scotland, aiding and abetting a suicide would probably not be a crime in Scotland. A physician who assists a patient to commit suicide in England may possibly be guilty under Section 2(1) of the Suicide Act 1961 although, as stated above, there is no evidence that this would happen. The authors suggest that a section should be added to the Suicide Act under Section 2 to the effect that a physician would be excluded from a charge if he or she was a registered medical practitioner who, given the existence of a competent directive, provided assistance to a patient who was suffering from a progressive and irremediable condition and who was prevented, or would be prevented, by physical disability from ending his or her own life without assistance.[15]

This bears a close resemblance to the conditions under which Dutch doctors have practised for a number of years, and it moves one step closer to mediating some of the thornier issues that have faced clinicians and the judiciary. Cases such as *Airedale NHS Trust v Anthony Bland*[5] would not necessarily have to be heard in court, but could be heard by multi-disciplinary panels of experts.

The information presented above has been fairly straightforward and factual, and this presents relatively few obstacles to a debate on euthanasia. The challenges arise when the philosophers and ethicists begin to present their arguments and counter-arguments. Who is right? As noted earlier, it is not possible to make a definitive statement about who is right or who is wrong, as each side will present a provocative debate. The task facing the student of ethics is to identify the sound arguments and those that are flawed. However, the greatest challenge of all is to recognise that no morally correct solution can be deduced from a single ethical principle. Having said this, some of the principles that may be used to guide us are inherently incompatible.[17] Some of us wish to debate in the hope that the decision will be less uncomfortable and the choices will be easier to make. Wishing it was so will not make it easier. However, believing that a balanced viewpoint and well-constructed thinking have been exercised in the discussion of this topic may assist us in feeling satisfied that all that could have been done was done. The following arguments have been heard in some form or another and at various levels of depth for many years. This brief summary provides the opportunity to identify an introduction to the argument surrounding euthanasia.

# The three components of a debate on euthanasia

Margaret Pabst Battin,[6] a bioethicist, identifies that it is a serious moral error to oppose euthanasia on the grounds of three fundamental moral principles, namely mercy, autonomy and justice.

The mercy argument has two essential components. Linked in a peripheral way to the double effect argument discussed below, is the principle of beneficence, which is seen as a duty to prevent or remove harm or a duty to promote good. This duty is best illustrated in palliative care as a duty to act to end pain or suffering that is already occurring. An alternative consideration to be held is that of non-maleficence – a duty not to do harm, which thereby forms a core of morality exhorting us not to cause further pain and suffering, not to kill, not to disable, and so on. These two elements, where healthcare professionals have a duty to balance the principles of beneficence and non-maleficence before making decisions about patient care, form the core of the mercy argument.

The healthcare professional might ask such questions as 'Is the treatment doing any good?', 'Is the treatment causing harm to the patient?' or 'Is the compliance with the patient's wishes harmful?' in order to determine the scope of intervention and treatment and to serve as a useful springboard for further discussions with the patient and their family. Thus euthanasia could be considered to be morally right. However, Rachels[18] develops this further into a more rigorous argument. He suggests that utilitarianism should be examined in the light of actions being right or wrong according to whether they caused happiness or misery. If the actions were judged by this standard, then euthanasia would be morally acceptable. The principle of utility states that any action is morally right if it increases the amount of happiness in the world or if it decreases the amount of misery. The argument then goes on to say that killing – at their own request – a terminally ill patient who is suffering intolerably would decrease the amount of suffering in the world, and therefore this action would be morally right. This argument, says Rachels, is much too simplistic to be entirely useful, as these are not the only morally important considerations. If this view is expanded to include the ability to maximise one's interests, then Rachels says that although the promotion of happiness and the avoidance of misery are not the only morally important issues, they are important nonetheless, so if an action decreases misery and suffering, then this is one very strong reason in its favour. The theme of incompatible ideals and ideas, and of more than one principle being applicable to the argument, is beginning to develop. Readers would be well advised to explore the doctrine of utilitarianism and the principle of utility further.

Those who are opposed to euthanasia say that the mercy argument is misplaced. Gormally[19] likens euthanasia to putting a sick or injured animal out of its misery – mercy is confused with loving care and wanting to do the best for the dying animal. He says that:

*mercy sustains and supports and you cannot take care of something by destroying it. But you can judge it not worth preserving, and sympathy is one of the things that can make it feel intolerable to put up with a creature's gross suffering and may even incline one to terminate a reduced and pathetic existence.*

This standpoint is supported by Brock,[20] who brings it within a more realistic framework. He says that the critical premise of the mercy argument is false because there are not great numbers of patients who are suffering, thanks to the advances of palliative care. If patients are suffering, he maintains, it is because there is a 'wrongful failure' to provide adequate pain relief. This is an interesting premise, and one on which the palliative care movement depends to actively oppose voluntary euthanasia. This will be discussed later in the chapter.

Another principle to be considered is that of autonomy, defined by Beauchamp and Childress[14] as 'a concept of self-governance: being one's own person, without constraint either by another's action or by psychological or physical limitations'. The autonomous person determines his or her own course of action in accordance with a plan chosen by him- or herself. Such a person deliberates about and chooses plans, and is capable of acting on the basis of such deliberations. Glover[3] states that questions of autonomy can only arise in the context of a person who has a preference at the time when a decision is to be taken, which then eliminates the mentally incompetent person from this arena. Faulder[21] states that at the very heart of autonomy is the concept of respect for persons and, by extension, a respect for the decisions that they choose to make and the rights that they choose to exercise. Pabst Battin[6] states that autonomy supports euthanasia:

> *one ought to respect a competent person's choices, where one can do so without undue costs to oneself, where doing so will not violate other moral obligations and where these choices do not threaten harm to any persons or parties.*

Pabst Battin suggests that if the threads of the arguments around mercy were picked apart, then every patient with an illness, injury or disability should be able to claim full support for whatever treatment they require, for as long as they require it. Can our society support such a concept? Can our financial and human resources stretch to infinity? Should resources be available to everyone, or only to a select few? Who would choose the few? Knowing that there have been some challenges to this notion, the principle of justice or fairness must be called into play to mediate and assist in distributing the limited resources that we have.

This is not a theoretical issue. Former British Secretary of State for Health, Virginia Bottomley, said that 'in a modern health service, every clinical decision took place within finite resources'.[22] This might include invoking justice based on the greatest medical need, or who can pay, or whether medical intervention would offer a complete restoration of function, or whose contributions to society have been the greatest. This principle can also assist with decisions to be made for those whose conditions are not self-induced (e.g. the non-smoker, or the person who does not abuse drugs). Pabst Battin states that it is often argued that if treatment is denied to people, with the result that they will die, then is it not better to deny treatment to those who are 'medically unsalvageable' and who will die in any case? This, she says, justifies the practice of euthanasia on the basis of what is known as the *salvageability principle* – salvaging those who will not die so soon and letting the others die (e.g. the terminally ill patient, the defective neonate). Euthanasia is in accord with this principle by the demands of justice in a situation of scarcity of resources. She does warn that denying treatment on the grounds of justice does not strictly qualify as euthanasia, as the denial of treatment is not undertaken in order to promote a 'good death'. Again this is a 'taster' for the reader who wishes to explore further the principles of distributive justice and to formulate personal arguments about its use.

Questions to ask might include 'Does justice provide a smokescreen for treatment-limiting decisions or passive euthanasia?', 'Does rationing present risks to our healthcare system?' or 'Which criteria might be used to justify euthanasia?'. There are many, many more questions to be asked, but not necessarily answered. The point is to identify many points of view so that balanced thinking and argument are the outcome.

One objection to the argument of justice is the 'slippery slope' argument, so called because it is argued that if we travel down the road of sanctioning euthanasia, then it is one further slide down the slippery slope to uncontrolled and unregulated action. There is widespread belief among philosophers and ethicists that the slippery slope argument is illogical and does not stand up to close scrutiny. The aim of this section is to equip the reader with an overview of critical thinking about the slippery slope argument. Again this is not an attempt to sway thinking, but is intended to allow the reader to develop a more balanced view of this rather persuasive argument.

Pabst Battin has identified four common errors of slippery slope thinking which all have the same feature in common – they are all unclear and rely on generalities to fuel the debate. The first error is that this line of reasoning fails to identify clearly what the bottom point of the slippery slope is or what it is that people fear most about the outcome of legalised euthanasia. Secondly, the cause of the slide down the slippery slope from the current situation to the predicted bad outcome is not identified. There are often obtuse references to impending wealth on the part of those who may benefit from the death of another, but this argument fails to identify clearly what the actual event is or has been.

The third flaw in the argument is that it does not demonstrate the badness of the outcome. As was seen in the previous argument, the bad outcome is never made clear. Pabst Battin states that:

*if the bad outcome is simply that any individual is recognised to have the right to die while the integrity of the decision to live or die were safeguarded, it is by no means clear that this would be a bad thing.*

There is another well-known argument that is used to fuel the euthanasia debate.

For those opposed to the practice of euthanasia, the Nazi practices during the Second World War inevitably enter into the discussion as an example of how the slippery slope has existed in the past. Rachels[18] offers a very clear and sound explanation of how this argument started and how it has been maintained for almost 50 years. The atrocities committed during the war by the Nazis against Jews and other 'undesirables', as they were then known, have been widely reported. The Nuremberg trials convicted several doctors of war crimes and of the atrocities committed during Hitler's regime.

The historical link between euthanasia and Nazism has been attributed to an American doctor, Leo Alexander, who identified an opportunity to use Nazi atrocities as a way to discredit euthanasia. He started by crafting a story that showed the Nazis as first using euthanasia as a way to assist the terminally ill. Once the first step was taken, so we are led to believe, the downward slide on the slippery slope was very easy – morals were abandoned and mass killing became easy. An article that Alexander wrote for the *New England Journal of Medicine* in 1949 stated that:

> *Whatever proportions [Nazi] crimes finally assumed, it became evident to all who investigated them that they started from small beginnings. The beginnings at first were merely a subtle shift in emphasis in the basic attitude of physicians. It started with the acceptance of the attitude, basic in the euthanasia movement, that there is such a thing as life not worthy to be lived. This attitude in its early stages concerned itself with the severely and chronically sick. Gradually the sphere of those to be included in this category was enlarged to encompass the socially unproductive, the ideologically unwanted, the radically unwanted and finally all non-Germans. But it is important to realise that the infinitely small wedged-in lever from which this entire trend of mind received its impetus was the attitude toward the non-rehabilitable sick.*[18]

Rachels offers us this rich historical account in order to set the stage for the other arguments that should counterbalance the Nazi argument on euthanasia. An implausible belief to be challenged is that Hitler and those involved in mass murders were initially altruistic individuals whose 'compassion' led them to kill out of a sense of mercy, and that it was this compassion that allowed them to carry on and commit the atrocities that have haunted us to the present day. Even the most uninformed reader would have difficulty believing that compassion could be so boundless, particularly in the knowledge of how much cruelty was involved in the commission of these acts.

The next issue to consider is that, in the context of this discussion, euthanasia is a voluntary request by a patient to bring about his or her death. Brock[20] identifies the need for opponents of euthanasia to consider that the values that are consistent with voluntary euthanasia are in no way consistent with the involuntary killing that defined the euthanasia of Hitler's concentration camps. In Nazi Germany there was never an element of consent on the part of the concentration-camp victims. There was no choice involved, no permission given. People were killed in the name of achieving the purity of the Aryan race. Rachels noted that Hitler accepted the notion of a life not worthy to be lived, but this was not the same notion that is accepted by those who are in favour of euthanasia today. Hitler's version of the life not worthy to be lived was the life that could not fulfil the dream of a pure race.

One of the final considerations in this counter-plan is to examine how Hitler used the word 'euthanasia' to add an element of respectability to his plan where no respectability would otherwise be ascribed. Rachels reminds us that when an action is performed that might otherwise be condemned, one way of hiding the true nature of that action is to invest it with a positive connotation. In other words, language is deliberately misused so as to confer a positive status on an abhorrent action. For Hitler, the use of the word 'euthanasia' implied that his actions and policies were much more benign than they actually were.

Tassano,[23] in his provocative style, challenges us further. He discards the dispute that philosophers have with this argument when they suggest that, in order for slippery slope thinking to occur, there must be commitment on our part to allow progression down the slippery slope, at least further than if we had allowed the first step to be taken. He maintains that the flaw in this argument is that the sequences that are predicted by invoking the slippery slope are not always merely imagined. He maintains that there are connections of social convention or of the law between them, and he believes that when legal restraints are removed, it is difficult to believe that we are not further down the slope. However, he maintains that the slippery slope argument is not sufficient to decide any one issue – for example, it cannot be used on its own to refute euthanasia. He exhorts us to remember that the slippery slope argument is not relevant. This is an invitation to read the many works on the subject in order to develop a balanced place for this argument in your own thinking.

Other detractors of the euthanasia debate suggest that the right to die brings with it a duty to kill, and that it becomes society's responsibility to provide the means by which this might happen. Is it possible that there will be a day in the future when terminally ill patients will sue their doctors for failing to kill them? Is this reversal of the slippery slope argument logical?

An ethical doctrine that is closely linked with passive euthanasia or 'treatment-limiting decisions' is the doctrine of double effect. A traditional Catholic doctrine, it suggests that 'one may perform an action with a bad effect – for instance, the death of a person – provided one foresees but does not *intend* (my italics) the bad effect; one must be doing the act to achieve a good effect'. As there can be two results from the single action, there is a double effect – hence the name of the doctrine.

The doctrine requires that four conditions are met. Firstly, the action must not be intrinsically wrong. Secondly, the person performing the act must intend only a good effect, not a bad one. Thirdly, the bad effect must not be the means of achieving the good effect. Finally, the good effect must be proportional to, or outweigh, the bad effect, according to Pabst Battin. The 1993 House of Lords report suggests the use of the term 'double effect' as it relates to the administration of drugs to relieve pain and suffering with the probable consequence that it will shorten someone's life, in preference to the term 'passive euthanasia'. The concept of intention is one that will not be explored further in this chapter, but it is worth examining in more extensive reading.

# The role of palliative care

A rich tradition of palliative care has developed around the world. One of the greatest fears shared by patients and members of their families is that they will experience a painful or otherwise distressing death. It has always been the mission of palliative care to relieve the symptoms of terminal illness, including pain, breathlessness and other distressing side-effects. Dame Cecily Saunders, one of the pioneering forces in the palliative care movement, said in 1972 that, 'All those who work with dying people are anxious that what is known already should be developed and extended and that terminal care everywhere should become so good that no one need ever ask for voluntary euthanasia.'[3]

Although there are some elements of this argument that can be supported, it is a fundamentally flawed thesis that fails to acknowledge some basic facts about the provision of palliative care and the underlying ability of an individual to choose their own destiny, regardless of what support is on offer.

As a general rule, the positive value of palliative care to the majority of patients and their carers cannot be denied. The level and quality of care generally provided help to alleviate many of the physical and psychological symptoms experienced by patients. As death is an unfamiliar experience to most people, it is likely that the treatments and support that are available to ameliorate this condition are not known to them. If a patient is part of a healthcare system that provides good palliative care and he or she is willing to accept it, then it is possible that some of the fears that would lead to him or her wanting to die prematurely could be allayed. However, palliative care – good or otherwise – is not equitably available. Where it is available, the bulk of effort and research has supported patients with cancer.

The benefits of good palliative care are vast, but it is too simplistic an argument to suggest that access to palliative care is the definitive answer for all patients who are at the end of their lives. A statistic quoted by the Nightingale Alliance, an anti-euthanasia lobbying organisation, states that with the aid of good palliative care, 95% of pain can be controlled and the remaining 5% can be made tolerable. If pain was the only issue at stake, this might be a compelling statistic. However, the people who have campaigned for or at least heightened the cause of assisted suicide have had motor neuron disease, and arguably their issues are different to those faced by the majority of cancer patients. Information in the popular press suggests that patients with motor neuron disease in particular voice frustration and concern at having to be cared for by someone else for many years, and about the fact that they have lost their independence. Palliative care is not a panacea, and however good the care, it may not be the answer for a select group of patients who do ask for a premature end to their lives. It is worth stressing that the number of patients who fall into this category is small.

It is still the case that specialist palliative care is an option for a relatively small number of patients who may fit into restricted diagnostic categories which include cancer, motor neuron disease and AIDS. The willingness or ability of the palliative care community to care for many patients outside these groups is still quite limited, due to either a lack of specialist clinical knowledge or the recognition that other diagnoses have a much less definable prognostic period which conflicts with the time-limited period that is often set by palliative care providers.

Weigands[24] suggests that patients in persistent vegetative state, for instance, would fall well outside the ambit of palliative care, as the perception is that they do not feel pain or necessarily experience any of the other symptoms that palliative care deals with so well.

Another flaw linked to this argument is the supposition that palliative care is so all-encompassing that it provides all of the answers to another person's suffering. Pabst Battin makes the powerful suggestion that not all pain or other distressing symptoms can be relieved by the best efforts of the palliative care community. She goes further to suggest that when this cannot occur, there are opportunities to sedate the patient into unconsciousness, thus ending the pain and symptoms. She maintains that this culminates in causing the patient's death with respect to the patient's experience. Linking in with the criteria of the proposed Medical Futility Bill, the patient has no further conscious experience and cannot experience significant communication. Pabst Battin concludes by saying:

> *Although it is always technically possible to achieve relief from pain, at least when the appropriate resources are available, the price may be functionally and practically equivalent, at least from the patient's view, to death. And this, of course, is what the issue of euthanasia is all about.*

Farsides[25] suggests that there may be a feeling of failure on the part of palliative care providers if a patient requests euthanasia. Those who provide palliative care have carved a niche for themselves as carers rather than curers, which in itself flies in the face of the traditional medical model. What the carers may not have reconciled themselves to, Farsides argues, is an acceptance of the way someone dies. At the bottom of a request for euthanasia is a perceived acknowledgement of failure on the part of the carers. How 'successful' a death is validates their ability. Far from validating a carer's needs, Farsides suggests that a request for euthanasia is an expression of personal autonomy. Regardless of the quality of care and the resources available to provide it, there are some individuals who are unable to countenance the thought of living with a deteriorating mind and/ or body. They may feel that being cared for is a burden which they are unable to live with. The argument is further and more powerfully developed by Ronald Dworkin,[26] who has suggested that 'a failure to acknowledge that someone wishes to die, or to die in a way that others approve, but that is a horrifying contradiction of the patient's life, is a devastating, odious form of tyranny'.

The ethical principles which have been under discussion have also found companion arguments that are commonly used to confirm the benefits or failings of euthanasia. When argued in the courts, there are arguments that arise time after time, almost as the practical disagreements that follow the theoretical ones. One such issue concerns the sanctity of life. Dworkin identifies the principle as the intrinsic value of life above all else. He states that it is the distinction between the intrinsic value of human life and its personal value for the patient that explains why so many people think euthanasia is wrong in all circumstances. It is at the heart of all religious arguments. John Locke, the philosopher, said that 'human life was not the property of the person living that life, who is just a tenant, but of God'. Dworkin goes on to say that the conviction of the sanctity of life provides a powerful emotional basis for euthanasia.

The conclusions reached by a working party on euthanasia and clinical practice in 1982 identified that:

> *men are not like other animals, they are spirit as well as flesh. Their lives are sustained by the power of God and at his will and, being spirit, a man can either consent or rebel against that will. . . . The valuation of human life is clearly religious ... a basically religious valuation of human life has preserved our homicide laws and has hitherto preserved us.*[27]

Is this a naive argument? Does opposition to euthanasia seem outmoded simply because it is a product of Christian teaching as James Rachels suggests? Does this mean that the non-religious person could find fault with the sanctity of life argument? Dworkin maintains that atheists may feel that human life has intrinsic value. This may identify the foundations for a profound argument that sanctity of life or the intrinsic value of life, whether secular or religious, are arguments for rather than against euthanasia.

Another argument that is put forward when considering the enormity of the subject of euthanasia is the 'best interests' argument. When thinking about other ethical principles that arise in palliative care, there are opportunities to examine the role of paternalism in decision making. Dworkin expands on this when he suggests that those who are opposed to euthanasia are opposed on paternalistic grounds – the decisions that they make are in the best interests of the patient. It is these individuals who know about the interests of the patient better than the patient. The problem with the best interests argument is that it is difficult to tell in whose best interests such decisions are made. The best interests argument has had a thorough airing in the British courts as, in particular, the House of Lords struggled with the decision to discontinue food and fluids for Tony Bland in *Airedale NHS Trust v Bland*.[5]

A healthcare professional or family member may feel that a patient does not need to know their diagnosis or prognosis, and the issue of 'truth-telling' becomes enmeshed in the best interests argument: Faulder[19] adds this to the list of ethical considerations, where it is known as the principle of veracity. Veracity is closely linked to trust, and if this is perceived as being abused by the patient, it is easy to see how the clinician–patient relationship could be eroded. 'Tell them what they need to know' and, particularly if it is something of a technical nature, 'assume that they will never understand it' seems to be a prevailing theme in paternalistic arguments. Perhaps not lie-telling, but at the least being economical with the truth and with information falls into this category. It is often unclear whether this is an altruistic approach that involves genuinely wanting to spare the patient the anxiety of dealing with the truth, or whether it is an issue of control. These are all areas to explore and reflect upon further.

A third argument is the substituted judgement test, often used in the courts when attempting to make decisions about the withdrawal of treatment for an incompetent patient, and in some cases on behalf of a competent patient. Unless the courts have a specific directive from a patient, such as an advance directive or 'living will' outlining definite choices with regard to treatment, they will (as they did in the case of Karen Quinlan) attempt 'to don the mental mantle' of the patient. In other words, the courts will attempt to identify through previous conversations and from a patient's former attitude to life what they would have chosen for themselves in terms of withholding or withdrawing treatment.

Two of the criticisms of this doctrine have been that it failed to differentiate between the competent and incompetent patient, and that it inferred competence where it may not have existed.[28] Advance directives have been developed to assist clinicians and the courts in more clearly identifying the wishes of a patient should they become mentally incompetent for whatever reason. In March 1995, the Law Commission published a report on mental incapacity recommending urgent reform in this area of the law, where it suggested that there should be statutory rules to clarify the law about the legality of advance statements or directives.

It should be noted that advance directives themselves are not necessarily dynamic documents. The individual who signs such a document does so knowing what technology and treatments are available at the time. An advance directive may 'expire' technologically due to advances in the field, and it is possible that there may be an efficacious treatment available later than was thought at the time of signing the document. It is for this reason that those who sign such documents should be vigilant about reviewing and revising their wishes on a regular basis. Following the groundwork laid by the most important legal case of this kind in the USA, namely the Karen Quinlan case cited earlier, a second PVS case refined the law regarding advance directives in the USA. *Cruzan v Director, Missouri Department of Health* played a very important role in assisting each State to make provision for advance directives. In 1990, Congress adopted a law requiring all federally supported hospitals to inform any admitted patient of each State's advance directive laws.

In contrast to the situation in the USA, physicians in England and Wales may find the directives 'helpful', but they are not bound to obey them.[17] Spiers identifies that they represent a beginning with regard to allowing a patient with specific wishes to reject treatment when they are no longer capable of articulating those wishes. There are real concerns that, at least in the UK and Canada, a doctor is not duty-bound under the law to respect a patient's wishes in an advance directive, and therefore a reliance on professional judgement that borders on the paternalistic comes into play. Tassano[23] suggests that the principal effect of these 'living wills' is to make it easier for doctors to withdraw treatments when they consider it appropriate, supporting the notion of paternalism.

The balance of all of these arguments is critical when examining the essential premises for discussions about euthanasia. Rights are central to the euthanasia debate. Rights can be moral or legal. A moral right must be proved to be grounded in universally applied principles and is intrinsically good. A moral right is not necessarily enforceable, although if sufficient public pressure exists, this may influence the drafting of legislation to protect that right. A legal right does not have to be supported by a moral principle – the only concern for the courts is what is right and what is wrong in the law.[21]

Do we have the right to ask for euthanasia? Who should be making these decisions? Should they continue to be discussed in the courts as criminal charges? Should these decisions be made only by healthcare professionals? Should there be non-judicial panels which will take the decisions out of the courts and place them in the hands of those who are 'at the coalface'?

These questions and many more are very real. If we are to be comfortable and credible when questions about the end of life are being discussed, we should be aware of all of the elements that are contained in the most often quoted principles. This chapter offers only a 'bird's-eye view' of the richness of the subject, and will certainly not fully inform any argument. Your role is to research and practise your arguments and beliefs. There is no right or wrong in this arena – this is your stage.

# References

1 Wilkes E (1994) On withholding nutrition and hydration in the terminally ill: has palliative medicine gone too far? A commentary. *J Med Ethics*. 20: 144.
2 Lamb D (1985) *Death, Brain Death and Ethics*. Avebury Press, London.
3 Glover J (1977) *Causing Death and Saving Lives*. Penguin Books, Harmondsworth.
4 Roy D and Rapin H (1995) Regarding euthanasia. *Eur J Palliat Med*. 1: 57–9.
5 House of Lords (1993) *Report of the Select Committee on Medical Ethics. Volume 1*. HMSO, London.
6 Pabst Battin M (1994) *The Least Worst Death*. Oxford University Press, Oxford.
7 American Medical Association (1996) Code of Medical Ethics: physician-assisted suicide. *Bulletin of Medical Ethics*. **June**: 6.
8 International Task Force on Euthanasia and Assisted Suicide (2003) *Five Years Under Oregon's Assisted Suicide Law*; www.internationaltaskforce.org/press1.htm.
9 Supreme Court of the United States of America, No. 04–623.
10 BBC News items; www.news.bbc.co.uk (28 November 2000, 1 April 2002, 24 December 2002).

11 Woodruff R (1999) *Euthanasia and Physician-Assisted Suicide: are they clinically necessary?*; www.hospicecare.com.

12 Nightingale Alliance; www.nightingalealliance.org/htmdocs/iss_e_j.htm.

13 Wright K (2000) Social Policy Section, House of Commons Library Research Paper. Medical Treatment (Prevention of Euthanasia) Bill 12 of 1999–2000; www.parliament.uk/commons/lib/research/rp2000/rp00-008.pdf.

14 Beauchamp TL and McCullough LB (1984) *Medical Ethics*. Prentice Hall, Englewood Cliffs.

15 Mason JK and Mulligan D (1996) Euthanasia by stages. *Lancet*. **347**: 810–11.

16 Medical Treatment (Prevention of Euthanasia) Bill. Research Paper 00/8. Bill 12 of 1999–2000, 24 January 2000. www.parliament.uk/commons/lib/rp2000/rp00-008.pdf.

17 Spiers J (1997) *Who Owns Our Bodies? Making moral choices in healthcare*. Radcliffe Medical Press, Oxford.

18 Rachels J (1986) *The End of Life: euthanasia and morality*. Oxford University Press, Oxford.

19 Gormally L (ed.) (1994) *Euthanasia, Clinical Practice and the Law*. Linacre Centre, London.

20 Brock D (1994) *Life and Death: philosophical ethics in biomedical ethics*. Cambridge University Press, Cambridge.

21 Faulder C (1985) *Whose Body Is It? The troubling issue of informed consent*. Virago Press, London.

22 Editorial (1995) Care in the courts. *The Times*. **11 March**.

23 Tassano F (1995) *The Power of Life and Death: a critique of medical tyranny*. Gerald Duckworth Ltd, London.

24 Weigands W (1988–89) Has the time come for Doctor Death? Should physician-assisted suicide be legalised? *J Health Law*. **7**: 321–50.

25 Farsides C (1996) Euthanasia: failure or autonomy? *Int J Palliat Nurs*. **2**: 102–5.

26 Dworkin R (1993) *Life's Dominion*. Harper Collins, London.

27 Linacre Centre (1984) *Report of a Working Party on Euthanasia: trends, principles and alternatives*. Linacre Centre, London.

28 Oxman M (1989–90) The encouragement of empathy: just decision making for incompetent patients. *J Law Health*. **3**: 189–217.

# Further reading

Davies M (1998) *Textbook on Medical Law* (2e). Blackstone Press, London.

Gormally L (ed.) (1994) *Euthanasia, Clinical Practice and the Law*. Linacre Centre, London.

Jones M (2001) *Textbook on Torts* (7e). Blackstone Press, London.

Kennedy I and Grubb A (2000) *Medical Law* (3e). Butterworth, London.

Law Commission Report (1995) *Mental Incapacity*. HMSO, London.

Sheldon T (1997) Dutch relax euthanasia rules. *BMJ*. **314**: 325.

Spanjer M (1996) Dutch euthanasia society solicits complaints. *Lancet*. **348**: 954.

Zinn C (1997) Australia repeals world's first right-to-die law. *The Guardian*. **25 March**.

# 8 Teaching ethics in the practice setting

## Rachel Burman

The importance of clinical ethics should not now be in doubt. It is based on the four basic prima facie principles of beneficence, non-maleficence, autonomy and justice. The expansion of the subject comes in the context of enormous advances (both technological and scientific) in the practice of medicine. With this has come an increasing public professional interest in its implications. The issue of limited resources and the open discussion of the allocation of those resources is now a matter of repeated public interest.

With this must also come a responsibility of healthcare workers to be educated in these principles and their application to the clinical setting.

Historically, the discussion of ethical issues in medicine took place primarily within the medical profession itself. The first and most often quoted ethical code, namely the Hippocratic oath, still the basis of the ethical code by which doctors are taught to practise, is the teaching of a physician, Hippocrates. But medical ethics is not a purely medical discipline. It is the fusion or merging of many disciplines – behavioural sciences, law, theology and philosophy as well as medicine. Thus modern bioethics is the synthesis of a multi-disciplinary, pluralist approach. Arguably, therefore, it seems that it is also best discussed and taught to multi-disciplinary groups. An understanding of the principles of bioethics is vital to all those involved in the education of healthcare workers to ensure that their own practice is defensible and justified ethically. It is also equally important in their role as teachers influencing healthcare workers in their learning and decision making, so that any decisions they should then subsequently make concerning their clients take on a justifiable ethical dimension.

Palliative care has as its core not only the discipline of rigorous control of pain and other symptoms, but also the need for patient-centred communication, the holistic care of the patient and their family, consideration of the needs of the patient in the context of their family, consideration of any advanced wishes of the patient, and respect for the spiritual or religious beliefs of the patient and their family. Underpinning this must be an ethical framework on which to base

**121**

decision making. Since its inception, palliative care has adopted and actively fostered the multi-professional approach to the total holistic care of patients. This model is one which palliative care has promoted to other healthcare disciplines, and this philosophy has relevance to much of healthcare generally. Palliative care has always had interests which cut across traditional departmental and divisional lines – it has adopted novel approaches to inter-departmental and inter-disciplinary programmes throughout its evolution. Palliative care is therefore well placed to again lead the field in the multi-disciplinary teaching of bioethics.

The practice of palliative care takes place within the whole spectrum of clinical or practice settings. There is the more traditional model of hospice-based work, this inpatient setting also offering an outreach facility through a home care team which works with the patient and their family in the setting of their own home. In this practice setting there is close liaison with colleagues in district nursing and general practice. More recently there has been the development of hospital-based support teams. Teams of nurses, doctors and hospital social workers, in conjunction with colleagues in the physiotherapy and occupational health departments, provide a palliative care input to patients while they are in hospital. The patients seen in hospital may be at an earlier stage in their illness than those traditionally seen in the hospice setting, and the role of the team in facilitating information about the prognosis is essential. Patients in this practice setting may find that their first point of contact with palliative care concerns the discussion of the transition of their care from a curative to a palliative approach. There are specific ethical issues surrounding this. The palliative care team may be called upon to become involved in the discussion of the issues relating to withdrawal of treatment from a patient in the acute hospital setting.

The day-to-day practice of palliative care continually involves the confrontation and discussion of ethical issues which require a pragmatic resolution in the work of all healthcare professionals. Daily decisions about the ongoing treatment of terminally ill patients and the degree of active intervention that should be undertaken are discussed and taken. Maintaining respect for the patient's autonomy is particularly challenging in the context of a request for euthanasia from either a patient or a carer. The need to handle sensitively a carer's or patient's request for disclosure or non-disclosure of information, particularly concerning the length of the prognosis, is a constant dilemma. The different philosophical approaches to the issues that surround death and dying which are encountered when practising in a multi-faith society are all routine issues for a palliative care team. This team has always included not only nurses and doctors, but also social workers, counsellors and chaplains.

It is therefore universally accepted that the teaching of ethics is desirable. The next concern is how this is to be most effectively achieved. All of the professional bodies responsible for the content of courses for healthcare workers agree that an ethics component is indicated, but they are not explicit about what it should contain. The training of doctors is overseen by the General Medical Council, which has decreed that ethics teaching should be part of the core curriculum for medical students, but leaves the content and organisation of the teaching to the individual medical schools.[1] Furthermore there is a lack of staff with any training in the subject available to teach it. Grant *et al.*[2] and later Seedhouse[3] observe that courses are taught by people with no philosophical background, and insufficient time is allowed for proper analysis of ethical problems. The emphasis should be on allowing sensitive listening to and discussion of experiences and ethical dilemmas, with philosophers and clinicians facilitating this. On average, the length of time allocated to the subject is 0.1% of all undergraduate teaching. Self[4] confirms that the teaching of ethics is often didactic, focusing on curriculum content and teaching methods to the exclusion of the contribution that the medial students themselves can make. A number of studies have looked at the level of ethical awareness of various groups prior to their differing forms of training. Self showed a resistance to ethical teaching among some medical students, who considered that in a multi-cultural society all belief structures should be afforded equal respect, and that formal instruction in ethics would represent a form of indoctrination.

Grundstein-Amando[5] found difficulties between the various groups of health-care professionals. Nursing students were more generally concerned to motivate their ethical reasoning by the fundamental of caring, whereas medical students were more motivated by the concept of patients' rights. Other researchers have looked at other rationales for the apparent differences between various groups. Gilligan[6] postulates that there is a difference based on gender, with women more often viewing morality in the context of particular relationships, whereas men sublimate this to a view of impartiality and justice. Kolhberg[7] disagrees with this construct, arguing that personal morality has little to do with gender and more to do with the individual. Nolan and Smith[8] showed that medical students do not come to their training devoid of material which could form the basis of a programme of ethics teaching. On the contrary, they have already derived much from relevant reading and work experience prior to attending medical school. Another finding of this study was that the majority of students considered the teaching of ethics to be important, and would like this teaching to be practically based.

There is a growing call for ethical teaching in the undergraduate curriculum, but there is not the corresponding attention to the subject in the clinical training years. Recent studies in the UK and the USA showed that practising physicians felt their education in treating disease was excellent, whereas areas such as healthcare resource allocation and ethical issues were poorly covered. These studies have highlighted barriers to change, such as departmentalisation of the medical school, lack of leadership and lack of faculty development. Despite recognition of the need for change there has been little substantial curricular innovation, and then only in the preclinical years. Fleischman and Arras[9] observed that the ad hoc discussion of cases without reference to philosophical principles tends to yield aimless, ungrounded speech. Conversely, abstract theoretical discussion of philosophical doctrines often proves irrelevant to the concrete and urgent concerns of the physician.

The challenge in teaching medical students is to integrate philosophical theory with concrete clinical case material. The special perspective of the family practitioner has been evaluated by Stevens *et al.*[10] This is an example of case-based teaching in the primary care setting. A sessional course meets weekly for ten sessions to discuss ethical topics such as truth-telling, informed consent and autonomy. The family practitioner then presents a real case from their practice and explains it up to the point when the ethical decision is made. At this point, the group of students is encouraged to discuss what decision they would reach. The goals of these sessions are to develop the students' abilities to define the issues and think about possible resolutions in a way that also helps them to analyse their own moral reasoning. These classes include not only medical students but also students of nursing, pharmacy and physiotherapy. The students reported that representations of different professional disciplines enriched the group, that the use of everyday clinical cases was much more instructive than the use of more highly published dilemmas, and that exposure to the family practitioner enabled them to understand context-sensitive care.

One model which has tried to cross the disciplines in its approach to the teaching of ethics in the clinical years is in practice at the University of California at Los Angeles (UCLA) medical school.[11] In the third year of study (i.e. the first clinical year), the students follow a longitudinal programme of simulated practice sessions in which they meet one or two patients and follow up three or four patients. These simulations use taped phone calls and video consultations with patients. The content of these encounters is built around 25 of the patient scenarios most commonly seen by a hospital doctor, and includes issues of ethics and resource allocation. Thus the students follow the course of these patients and, in ordering their tests and discussing their management, gain experience of evidence-based medicine. By participating in the small discussion groups through the year they become confident in the reasoning needed to explore the ethical issues that are encountered in clinical practice. This model of training has the benefit of integrating the ethical teaching into the clinical situation in a realistic and therefore accessible way for the students, who report that it has been much easier to see the relevance of this subject to their work as doctors. This contrasts with the complaints of other students that in their experience ethical teaching is didactic and too philosophical.

Joseph and Conrad[12] have published research looking specifically at the issue of ethical training in social work. They rightly argue that for the effective working of the multi-professional team, a social worker must feel confident to participate in the team's discussion of ethical dilemmas. They also point out that, to date, there has been little formal training available. The absence of this ability will, in time, lead to abdication of moral power and diminished professional responsibility. Further work by Joseph and Conrad identifies some predictors of social work influence in this area. They emphasise the ethical dilemmas pertaining not only to the client but also to the inter-professional issues of skill mix, information sharing and role clarity. They also have the courage to challenge the quality of the people who are currently responsible for what teaching there is. They highlight the fact that there is not necessarily adequate preparation of the professionals who are given this responsibility.

Several authors[13,14] have expressed the view that the nursing body is the one best able to move into the arena of bioethics. They argue that nurses are equipped with a large amount of clinical experience and are the professionals most likely to deal with the day-to-day manifestations of ethical dilemmas and the patients and families that those dilemmas affect. There has long been a tradition of nurses putting themselves forward as the patient and family advocate. This tradition sits well with the basic principle of respect for patient autonomy. Nurses also more often than other healthcare workers return to structured further study following a period of clinical work. The scene is therefore set for the synthesis of practical experience and more formal philosophical thought and teaching, which is agreed to form the necessary basis for bioethics. This discipline is about the personal side of healthcare as it deals with settling or preempting possible conflicts between professional medical expertise and the autonomy of the patient and their family. Some would argue that nurses are best placed for this role, once they have been trained in ethical principles and reasoning.

A recent development in the application of medical ethics is the formation of ethical committees[15] and, most recently of all, the concept of an ethical consultation with an ethicist. This practice is still confined to the USA and Canada, where many of the larger hospitals have resident ethicists on their staff. Ethical commit-tees in this context are not the same as those in the UK, which are solely for the consideration of research protocols submitted in the hospital setting. In the USA, ethics committees are commonplace in healthcare institutions. They have a multi-professional membership, with equal numbers of physicians and nurses together with members who are lawyers, clergy, social workers, administrators, members of the public and patients. The process of membership selection is not always clearly set out, but is based on some past experience and the ability to contribute to the committee. These committees normally have a threefold purpose, namely the recommendation of policy, a role in the education of healthcare professionals in the hospital, and a role in specific case consultations. Many of the policies developed over the last ten years regarding such issues as Do Not Resuscitate orders and the usefulness of advance directives have been derived from the consensus of such committees. However, the existence of these committees and the formulation of their policies do not translate directly into the understanding of the clinicians themselves. There is often a gap between prevailing guidelines and the knowledge and views of many doctors and nurses. Following the creation of such policies, committees must create strategies to influence the atti-tudes of clinicians.

The role of education is pivotal to the successful implementation of these policies. An increase in healthcare practitioners' awareness of and ability to assess ethical problems will eventually ease the burden of the educational compo-nent to the work of the committee. Those committees that monitor the impact of the teaching on new professionals will also be able to help new schools and programmes. In addition, they will be able to influence the content of other modules that are being developed in other settings.

Specific case consultations are generally conducted by a team consisting of some members of the committee. Each team within the committee takes it in turns to be on call for a two-week period. There may be an addition to the team, based on a needs assessment and the area of expertise required. For example, in an issue concerning maternal–child matters, a member from the obstetrics team would be co-opted. On occasion, new members of the committee will attend in order to gain experience as observers. A request for a consultation may be made by a nurse, doctor or social worker, for example, or by the family or patient themselves. Most of the consultations take place within 48 hours of the referral being made. Normally a team leader is appointed and they will conduct the consultation.

The first objective is to delineate the problems of the particular case, which are often the result of a lack of communication between the healthcare team and the patient. The emphasis is not on the ethical knowledge of the team, but more on what the team can enable or mediate for the patient and their family.

There are a number of questions which need to be addressed by the team. These include whether the patent is competent, the belief system of the patient, whether there are any particular requests or mandates that the patient wants to make, and what (if any) conflicts there are between the health professional and the patient.

Following this process the issues are summarised and the patient and their family make decisions which are then looked at by the team from an ethical perspective. Group consensus is usually achieved. This approach not only clarifies the values and explores the ethical dilemmas, but also allows a decision to be made.

In the USA, this model of ethical teaching and practice is being extended to the community setting. This committee process, which started as a self-educating one, is now increasingly expanding its educational efforts to healthcare workers and the public. It is also increasingly expanding its efforts in the area of healthcare resource allocation.[16]

In conclusion, it can be seen that all healthcare professionals, of whatever discipline, recognise a need for the inclusion of ethical reasoning in their respective training. It is also clear that this is pertinent to the specialty of palliative care. A review of the literature has shown that what healthcare professionals bring even at the point of beginning their respective training has a bearing on the way that they most effectively learn these principles and the reasoning skills necessary to apply them.

Some authors have rightly raised the issue of who is best placed to teach this subject, to whom and with whom. The literature supports the principle of interdisciplinary teaching and learning, suggesting that the cross-fertilisation of this approach is beneficial to all. This is a concept that fits well with the teaching that take place on other topics and the specialty of palliative medicine, and it can readily be adopted and built upon by all healthcare workers in the discipline.

It has been shown that the quality of the teaching given to students is in itself necessary to validate the subject of medical ethics and to emphasise its obvious importance. Although it seems to be universally accepted that the theoretical teaching of medical ethics has a place early on in the curricula of all healthcare workers, the teaching is often didactic in nature. The need for it to be contextualised in the clinical setting with the use of case histories is not always recognised, and the teaching is therefore less effective. Not surprisingly, the teaching and unfortunately the subject itself are then valued less highly. This is especially true of the experience of medical students at present. The evolution of ethical committees and the formalising of the ethical consultation highlight the fact that the best practice is that of multi-professional working.

Palliative care in the UK is already well established in its practice of multi-professional teamworking, and should therefore more easily adopt this effective approach when dealing with the ethical dilemmas that are encountered and teaching these principles to other healthcare workers – either in training or already practising.

# References

1 General Medical Council (1993) *Tomorrow's Doctors: recommendations for under-graduate medical education*. General Medical Council, London.
2 Grant VJ *et al.* (1989) Advanced medical ethics for fifth-year students. *J Med Ethics*. **15**: 200–2.
3 Seedhouse D (1991) Healthcare ethics teaching for medical students. *Med Educ*. **25**: 230–7.
4 Self DJ (1988) The pedagogy of two different approaches to humanistic medical education: cognitive vs affective. *Theor Med*. **9**: 227–36.
5 Grundstein-Amando R (1992) Differences in ethical decision-making processes among nurses and doctors. *J Adv Nurs*. **17**: 129–37.
6 Gilligan C (1982) *In a Different Voice*. Harvard University Press, Cambridge, MA.
7 Kohlberg L (1971) From is to ought. In: T Mitchel (ed.) *Cognitive Development and Epistemology*. Academic Press, New York.
8 Nolan PW and Smith J (1995) Ethical awareness in first-year medical, dental and nursing students. *Int J Stud*. **32**: 506–17.
9 Fleischman AR and Arras J (1987) Teaching medical ethics in perinatology. *Clin Perinatol*. **14**: 395–402.
10 Stevens NG and McCormick TR (1993) Bringing the special perspective of the family physician to the teaching of clinical ethics. *J Am Board Fam Pract*. **7**: 38–43.
11 Slavin SJ, Wilkes MS and Usatine MD (1995) Doctoring ill: innovations in education in the clinical years. *Acad Med*. **70**: 1091–5.
12 Joseph MV and Conrad AP (1983) Teaching social work ethics for contemporary practice: an effective evaluation. *J Soc Work Educ*. **19**: 56–68.
13 Leavitt FJ (1996) Educating nurses for their role in bioethics. *Nurs Ethics*. **3**: 40–51.
14 Scott PA (1996) Ethics education and nursing practice. *Nurs Ethics*. **4**: 53–6.
15 Dunn AP and Hansen-Flaschen J (1994) Framework for analysing an ethical problem and conducting an ethical consultation. *Semin Nurs Manag*. **2**: 27–30.
16 Perlin T (1992) *Clinical Medical Ethics Cases in Practice*. Little, Brown and Co. Boston.

# Index